NEUROLOGY -
LABORATORY AND CLINICAL RESEARCH DEVELOPMENTS

THE SECONDARY INSULTS AFTER ICH

FROM MECHANISMS TO CLINICAL TRANSLATION

NEUROLOGY - LABORATORY AND CLINICAL RESEARCH DEVELOPMENTS

Additional books in this series can be found on Nova's website under the Series tab.

Additional e-books in this series can be found on Nova's website under the eBooks tab.

NEUROLOGY -
LABORATORY AND CLINICAL RESEARCH DEVELOPMENTS

THE SECONDARY INSULTS AFTER ICH

FROM MECHANISMS TO CLINICAL TRANSLATION

GAIQING WANG

NOVA BIOMEDICAL

New York

Library of Congress Cataloging-in-Publication Data

Library of Congress Control Number: 2016952366

ISBN: 978-1-63485-642-3

Published by Nova Science Publishers, Inc. † New York

CONTENTS

PREFACE

Intracerebral hemorrhage (ICH) is a type of acute stroke characterized by extravasation of blood into brain parenchyma and formation of hematoma, leading to edema and tissue damage in the brain. During ICH, rapid accumulation of blood within brain parenchyma leads to disruption of normal anatomy and increased local pressure. Depending on the dynamic of hematoma expansion, the primary damage occurs within minutes to hours from the onset of bleeding and is primarily the result of mechanical damage associated with the mass effect, which compress adjacent tissues, thus destroying them. The 'mass effect' is an important factor in the pathogenic events in ICH. But it is impossible to predict the events and it is difficult to intervene its mass effect. Secondary injury following ICH occurs with the development of hematoma (hematoma expansion), edema, free radical formation, inflammation, and direct cellular toxicity due to the deposited hematoma and subsequent degradation byproducts (Wang 2014). So understanding the mechanisms of secondary insults and hematoma expansion then finding the potential approaches to treat and prevent its occurance is important for patients with potential hematoma expansion. As a consequence of ICH, blood components enter brain parenchyma causing progressive damage to the surrounding brain. Unless hematoma is cleared, the reservoirs of blood continue to inflict injury to neurovascular structures and blunt the brain repair processes. So seeking and defining effective hematoma scavenger markers which can be intervened appropriately is meaningful for patients with ICH. As noted above, all which may contribute to improve outcomes in patients suffering from ICH.

ABSTRACT

Intracerebral hemorrhage (ICH) is an often fatal type of stroke. If the patient survives the ictus, the resulting hematoma within brain parenchyma triggers a series of adverse events causing secondary insults and severe neurological deficits. The secondary insults after ICH mainly results from hematoma components toxicity and hematoma expansion. So treatment with blood toxicity, prevention from hematoma expansion and the timely removal of hematoma are essential to reduce deleterious pathological process and improve clinical outcomes in patients suffering from ICH. This work divided into 3 chapters. In chapter 1, the mechanisms of secondary brain insults after ICH are discussed and key aspects associated with the oxidative stressand inflammation resulted from hematoma toxicity are outlined, then the coresponding interventionsare introduced; In chapter 2, available information of hematoma expansion from clinical signs to molecular mechanisms are provided and potential intervention strategies discussed. Accumulating evidences suggest that multiple clinical markers such as coagulation/hemostasis dysfunction, higher blood pressure and BRAIN scores, higher serum glucose and/or glycosylated hemoglobin A1c, serum creatinine, Factor XIII and international normalized ratio (INR), lower serum cholesterol or LDL cholesterol, and fibrinogen, may be correlated with incidents of hematoma expansion. Furthermore, activation of several molecular pathways (i.e., plasma kallikrein, von Willebrand factor, N-methyl-D-aspartate and its receptor, cytokines/ adipokines, cellular fibronectin and apolipoprotein Eε2 allele) may lead to hematoma expansion. In chapter3, theendogenous hematoma scavenging system and potential intervention strategiesto facilitate hematoma resolution are discussed. Endogenous garbage cleaning system also known as scavenger receptors play important roles in the regulation of hematoma resolution in ICH. We try toillustrate how the endogenous garbage-cleaning system or scavenger receptors system in the brain work together to remove blood from the brain and reduce secondary brain insults, and presents potential clinically relevant molecular targets that could be harnessed to speed up this process via the endogenous phagocytosis. Meanwhile, guidelines of recommendations for clinical management of ICH are provided.

Keywords: intracerebral hemorrhage, secondary insults, hematoma expansion, clinical signs, biomarkers, molecular indexes, hematoma resolution, phagocytosis, scavenger receptors, clinical strategies

METHODS

In Chapter 1, we searched MEDLINE and GOOGLE with the keywords "Secondary Insults and Intracerebral Hemorrhage/Cerebral Hemorrhage/Brain Hematoma," "Secondary Injury and Intracerebral Hemorrhage/Cerebral Hemorrhage/Brain Hematoma," "Secondary Damage and Intracerebral Hemorrhage/Cerebral Hemorrhage/Brain Hematoma," "Inflammation and Intracerebral Hemorrhage/Cerebral Hemorrhage/Brain Hematoma," "Oxidative Stress and Intracerebral Hemorrhage/Cerebral Hemorrhage/Brain Hematoma." We excluded hemorrhage from SAH, aneurysm and trauma.

In Chapter 2 (Wang and Zhang 2016), We searched MEDLINE and GOOGLE with the keywords "Hematoma Expansion," "Hematoma Enlargement," "Hematoma Growth," "Rebleeding," "Secondary Bleeding," "Recurrent Bleeding" and "Rehemorrhage." We excluded hemorrhage from SAH, aneurysm and trauma.

In Chapter 3, we searched MEDLINE and GOOGLE with the keywords "Hematoma Resolution," "Hematoma Absorption," "Hematoma clearance," "Hematoma removal," "Hematoma Scanvenge," "Hematoma Evacuation," "Hematoma Phagocytosis," "Garbage Cleaning System," "Scavenger Receptors," "Erythrophagocytosis," "Blood Degradation Products" and "PPARγ Agonist."

Articles were selected for their conceptual importance and primacy. Where issues are controversial, evidence on both sides of the issue is given.

Chapter 1

THE SECONDARY INSULTS AND INTERVENTIONS FOLLOWING INTRACEREBRAL HEMORRHAGE: CURRENT UNDERSTANDING

ABSTRACT

Following intracerebral hemorrhage (ICH) the toxicity of extravasated blood plasma components including blood derived coagulation factors, complement components, immunoglobulins and other bioactive molecules are proposed to act as contributors to ICH-affected tissue damage. Subsequently, red blood cell (RBC) lysis starts at approximately 24h and continues for the next several days, leading to release of cytotoxic hemoglobin (Hb) with further deterioration of the pathological status quo. Hb and its degradation products, heme and iron, directly compromise the well-being of neighboring brain cells. Hb and heme are potent cytotoxic chemicals capable of causing death to many brain cells. Prominently, the mechanism of Hb toxicity is via generating free radicals (mainly through Fenton-type mechanism) and massive oxidative damage to proteins, nucleic acids, carbohydrates and lipids. Therefore, finding means of controlling inflammation, and detoxification, and absorption of Hb, heme and iron may have important clinical implications. In this chapter, the mechanisms of secondary brain insults after ICH are discussed and key aspects associated with the oxidative stress and inflammation resulted from hematoma toxicity are outlined, then the corresponding interventions (surgery and nonsurgery approaches)are introduced.

INTRODUCTION

Intracerebral hemorrhage (ICH) is a devastating form of stroke associated with a high rate of morbidity and mortality. After ICH the extravasated blood components (primarily erythrocytes and plasma proteins) and the "damage"-associated molecular patterns (DAMPs), impose a strong cytotoxic, pro-oxidative and pro-inflammatory insult toward adjacent viable brain cells, and could be seen as early as minutes after onset of ICH. It is now believed that much of this damage occurs in the subacute period following the initial insult via a cascade of complex pathophysiologic pathways that continues to be investigated. Increased levels of certain serum proteins have been identified as biomarkers that may reflect or directly participate in the inflammation, blood brain barrier disruption, endothelial dysfunction, and neuronal and glial toxicity that occur during this secondary period of cerebral injury. Some of these biomarkers have the potential to serve as therapeutic targets or surrogate endpoints for future research or clinical trials. So much work remains to be done, biomarkers show significant potential to expand clinical options and improve clinical management, thereby reducing mortality and improving functional outcomes in ICH patients (Aronowski and Zhao 2011).

1. CURRENT UNDERSTANDING OF THE MECHANISMS UNDERLYING ICH-INDUCED BRAIN INJURY

During intracerebral hemorrhage (ICH), rapid accumulation of blood within brain parenchyma leads to disruption of normal anatomy and increased local pressure. Depending on the dynamic of hematoma expansion (growth), the primary damage occurs within minutes to hours from the onset of bleeding and is primarily the result of mechanical damage associated with the mass effect (Qureshi, Mendelow et al. 2009). Secondary damage is for the most part due to the presence of intraparenchymal blood may be dependent upon the initial hematoma volume, age or ventricular volume, and it may occur through many parallel pathological pathways including: (1) cytotoxicity of blood, (2) hypermetabolism, (3) excitotoxicity, (4) spreading depression, (5) oxidative stress and inflammation. Ultimately, this pathogenesis leads to irreversible disruption of the components of the neurovascular unit, constituting gray and white matter, and is followed by blood-brain-barrier disruption and deadly brain edema with massive brain cell death. While inflammatory mediators generated locally in response to brain death/injury have the capacity to augment damage caused by ICH (secondary injury), the involvement of inflammatory cells e.g., microglia/macrophages is vital for removal/cleanup of cellular debris from hematoma, the source of ongoing inflammation (Aronowski and Zhao 2011). Primary and secondary brain damage after intracerebral hemorrhage was illustrated in Figure 1.

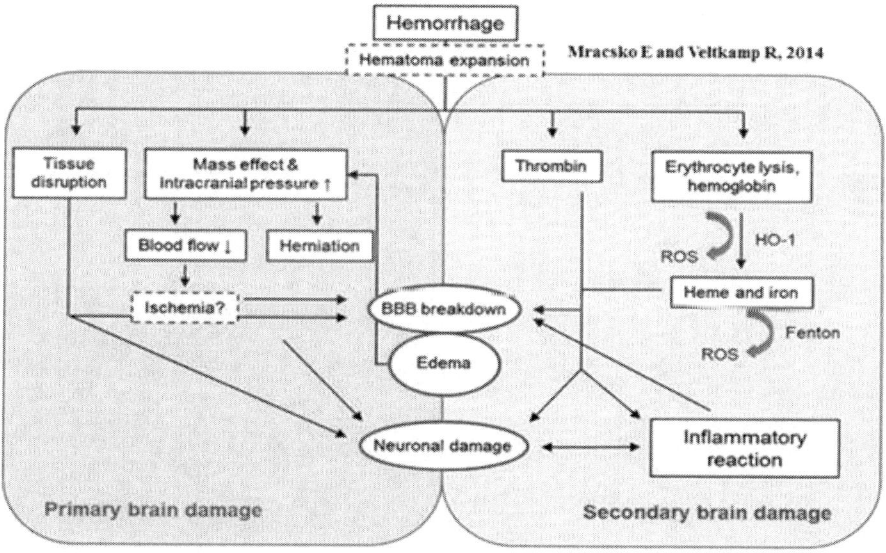

Figure 1. Primary and secondary brain damage after intracerebral hemorrhage.

Brain injury due to ICH initially occurs within the first few hours as a result of mass effect due to hematoma formation. But many patients continue to deteriorate clinically despite no signs of rehemorrhage or hematoma expansion. This continued insult after primary hemorrhage is believed to be mediated by direct toxicity and inflammatory responses induced by the components and metabolic products of late-stage hematomas and aggravates neurologic deficits (Keep, Hua et al. 2012). In other words, besides the mechanical tissue damage caused by the initial hematoma, injured brain cells and the extravasated components of the blood clot trigger a complex sequence of parallel and sequential deleterious mechanisms including inflammatory and oxidative stress pathways (Mracsko and Veltkamp 2014). It also said intracerebral blood itself has "toxic" effects beyond its mass effect (Xi, Wagner et al. 1998). Brain edema formation following ICH appears to be partly related to erythrocyte lysis and hemoglobin (Hb) release. Oxidative stress caused by components of the lysed erythrocytes contributes to the brain injury after ICH (Wu, Hua et al. 2002). Hb, heme, and iron released after red blood cell lysis aggravate ICH-induced severe brain edema and direct neuronal damage. Therefore, neutralization of Hb, heme and iron could represent an important target for reducing the secondary injury after ICH (Xi, Keep et al. 2006, Hua, Keep et al. 2007, Thiex and Tsirka 2007, Zhao, Song et al. 2011, Caliaperumal, Ma et al. 2012, Ding, Chen et al. 2014, Lakovic, Ai et al. 2014, Xiong, Wang et al. 2014). The major factors contributing to brain injury after ICH were shown in Figure 2.

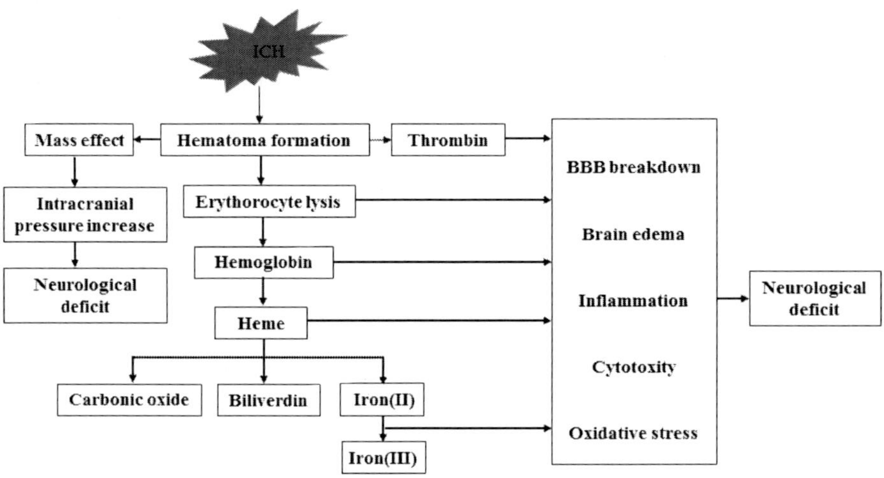

Figure 2. Mechanism of brain injury after ICH.

At this early stage the toxicity of extravasated blood plasma components including blood derived coagulation factors, complement components, immunoglobulins and other bioactive molecules are proposed to act as contributors to ICH-affected tissue damage. Subsequently, red blood cell (RBC) lysis starts at approximately 24h and continues for the next several days, leading to release of cytotoxic hemoglobin (Hb) with further deterioration of the pathological status quo (Wagner, Sharp et al. 2003). Hb and its degradation products, heme and iron, directly compromise the well-being of neighboring brain cells (Peeling, Yan et al. 1998, Wagner, Sharp et al. 2003, Wu, Hua et al. 2003, Zhao, Song et al. 2009, Wang, Manaenko et al. 2016). Hb and heme are potent cytotoxic chemicals capable of causing death to many brain cells (Wang, Manaenko et al. 2016). Prominently, the mechanism of Hb toxicity is via generating free radicals (mainly through Fenton-type mechanism) and massive oxidative damage to proteins, nucleic acids, carbohydrates and lipids (Qing, Dong et al. 2009, Wang, Yang et al. 2011, Wang, Hu et al. 2015, Wang, Shao et al. 2015). Therefore, finding means of controlling hemolysis, and detoxification, and absorption of Hb, heme and iron (Figure 1) may have important clinical implications (Aronowski and Zhao 2011).

1.1. Thrombin

Activation of hemostatic mechanisms is a physiological tissue response to hemorrhage to stop the bleeding. Thrombin, a serine protease produced rapidly after ICH onset, plays a pivotal role in the blood coagulation cascade. In response to bleeding, a complex series of clotting-factor interactions leads to its conversion by thromboplastin to thrombin, which transforms fibrinogen in plasmainto fibrin, as well as catalyzing many other coagulation-related reactions. As part of its activity in the coagulation cascade, thrombin also promotes platelet activation and aggregation via activation of protease-activated receptors on the cell membrane of the platelet (Wang 2014). Thrombin is essential for the blood coagulation processes and gets activated within the first hour after ICH (Gong, Xi et al. 2008). The primary purpose of thrombin is to stop bleeding as soon as possible and prevent hematoma expansion. Besides its physiological role, substantial lines of evidence indicate that thrombin participates in various pathological conditions in the brain, which contributes to edema formation and blood–brain barrier damage in early brain injury, and activates the cytotoxic, excitotoxic and inflammatory pathways that are involved in secondary injury following ICH. In the case of ICH, a large amount of blood-derived thrombin invades the brain tissue and exerts biological actions through its proteolytic activity. The substrates for thrombin include proteinase-activated receptors that transduce intracellular signals via trimeric G proteins. The role of thrombin in ICH pathogenesis was first suggested by its possible involvement in edema formation. That is, injection of whole blood into the striatum of rats induced edema, which was prevented by addition of hirudin, a thrombin inhibitor. Edema induced by autologous blood injection into the striatum was attenuated also by argatroban, another inhibitor of thrombin, even when the drug was systemically administered from 6 h after blood injection. ICH-associated edema results from disruption of the blood–brain barrier and death of brain parenchymal cells, both of which may be induced by thrombin. Application of thrombin to rat corticostriatal cultures induced delayed neuron death in the cortical region and shrinkage of the striatal region. Various pharmacological examinations revealed distinct properties of the mechanisms of injury between the cerebral cortex and the striatum. For example, extracellular signal-regulated kinase (ERK), p38, and c-Jun N-terminal kinase (JNK), three major members of mitogen-activated protein kinase (MAPK) family, all contributed to thrombin-induced injury of the striatum, whereas ERK, but not p38 or JNK, was involved in cortical injury. In addition, depletion of microglia from slice cultures rescued striatal tissue, but not cortical cells, from thrombin-induced injury, suggesting that microglia participate only in striatal tissue injury. Involvement of MAPKs and activated microglia in striatal tissue injury was confirmed by an in vivo study where thrombin was directly injected into the striatum of adult rats. On the other hand, plasminogen was found to cooperate with thrombin in inducing cortical injury but not striatal injury. Thrombin-mediated cellular injury may also be mediated by activation of matrix metalloproteinase (MMP)-9. That is, concurrent application of MMP-9 exacerbates cytotoxicity of thrombin in neurons in primary culture, and thrombin cytotoxicity is partially attenuated by MMP inhibitors. Moreover, brain damage induced by autologous blood injection is synergistically attenuated by deletion of the gene encoding MMP-9 and administration of the thrombin inhibitor hirudin. Intracerebral injection of thrombin leads to early brain edema formation by direct opening of the BBB and to neuronal damage at days 1 and 3 after ICH. High concentrations of thrombin induce neuronal damage in vitro, however, low concentrations are neuroprotective against various insults including ischemia or oxidative stress. Moreover, thrombin has an important role in brain recovery after intracerebral hemorrhagepossibly via the initiation of neurogenesis and angiogenesis (Aronowski and Zhao 2011). So, Thrombin can be a double-edged sword, It should be protective during the early stage inICH to rapidly stop bleeding and prevent hematoma enlargement , whereas its augment in the late stage may result in edema formation and be toxic (Wang 2014).

1.2. Inflammatory Cells/Meditors

Once ICH occurs, the hematoma gradually dissociated and released its components, such as hemoglobin (Hb), heme, iron, etc., into the perihematoma tissues. Then, these components of hematoma immediately trigger the inflammatory responses, which subsequently recruit and activate most inflammatory cells involved in the brain inflammatory injury. For example, the activated resident microglia and astrocyte, releasing a large amount of proinflammatory cytokines such as interleukin (IL)-6, TNF-α, and IL-1β, are in response to the blood components implicated in the initial brain injury after ICH. This inflammatory cascade leads to more neuron death;meanwhile, the dead neurons release the dangerassociated molecular patterns (DAMPs), such as highmobility group protein box-1 (HMGB1), to recruit more inflammatory cells infiltration into the brain, which further aggravates inflammatory brain damage (Xiong and Yang 2015).

Inflammation is characterized by the accumulation and activation of inflammatory cells and mediators within the hemorrhagic brain. ICH allows the immediate infiltration of blood components, including red blood cells, leukocytes, macrophages, plasma proteins, etc, into the injury site. The inflammatory response that follows this infiltration involves inflammatory mediator release, protease activation, microglia and astrocyte activation, brain tissue breakdown, and repair (Wang 2010). Increasing evidence has shown that inflammation is the key contributor of ICH-induced secondary brain injury. Inflammation progresses in response to various stimuli produced after ICH. Hematoma components initiate inflammatory signaling via activation of microglia, subsequently releasing proinflammatory cytokines and chemokines to attract peripheral inflammatory infiltration. Preclinical studies have identified inflammatory signaling pathways that are involved in microglial activation, leukocyte infiltration, toll-like receptor (TLR) activation, and danger associated molecular pattern regulation in ICH (Zhou, Wang et al. 2014). Toll-like receptor 4-mediated nuclear factor kappa-B signaling mediates the activation and regulation of inflammatory responses in the hemorrhagic brain and could be a therapeutic target for ICH (Wang 2010). Neuroinflammation is recognized as a vital factor in the pathophysiology of ICH-induced brain injury and is characterized by microglia activation, leukocyte infiltration, and cytokine and chemokine production. In addition to the release of inflammatory factors, the activation of inflammatory cells following ICH, initially to remove oxidative toxins, also participates in ROS production (Hu, Tao et al. 2016). Inflammatory cells include blood-derived leukocytes and macrophages, resident microglia, astrocytes, and mast cells (Wang 2010). A recent human ICH study that used microarray analysis demonstrated significant up-regulation of both pro- and anti-inflammatory genes in the peri-ICH brain tissue, a finding consistent with the results of a previous animal study. Little data regarding ICH pathogenesis have been obtained from postmortem human brain, and more studies are critically needed (Wang 2010).

1.2.1. Microglias/Macrophages Activation

Microglias are the primary immune effector cells in the brain and are often referred to as the brain's macrophages. In normal brains, resting microglia exhibit ramified morphology and constitute approximately 5–20% of the total glial population. The processes and protrusions of microglia have been observed to interact dynamically with neighboring neurons, astrocytes, and blood vessels. In response to various types of brain damage, microglia become activated (also referred to as reactive) and undergo morphologic and functional transformations. Specifically, the cell body becomes enlarged with thick processes, pro-inflammatory proteins are upregulated, and the cells become migratory, proliferative, and phagocytotic. Activated microglia are believed to have both neurotoxic and neuroprotective properties. The overall effect depends on pathologic conditions and brain injury severity (Wang 2010).

Activated microglia/macrophages can be identified by microscopy. Both resting and activated microglia/macrophages can be visualized by immunohistochemistry, and activated cells can be easily identified by their hypertrophic morphology. Accumulating evidence indicates that microglia/macrophages are activated early after ICH and that this activation contributes to ICH-induced secondary brain injury. After ICH, reactive microglia appear rod-like, spherical, or amoeboid, with short, strong processes, intense immunoreactivity, and a cell body usually more than 7.5 μm in diameter. In contrast, resting microglia are characterized by small cell bodies with a diameter less than 7.5 μm, ramified processes, and mild immunoreactivity. Although the major role for microglia/macrophages after ICH is to clear the hematoma and the tissue debris, reactive microglia/macrophages also express and release a variety of potentially toxic factors, such as cytokines, chemokines, ROS, proteases, cyclooxygenase-2, prostaglandins, and HO-1 and its metabolites. In addition, the degree of microglia/macrophage activation has been shown to be greater in aged rats after ICH than in young rats. It remains unclear how to differentiate activated microglia from macrophages recruited from the circulation (Wang 2010).

Many studies have suggested that activated microglia/macrophages contribute to ICH-induced early brain injury. Activation of microglia occurs much earlier than infiltration of neutrophils in and around the hematoma after collagenase-induced ICH (Wang 2010); the former occurs within 1 h, whereas the latter occurs after 4–5 h. The early response of microglia after ICH is consistent with the observation that focal microglia are activated immediately after BBB disruption by laser lesions. The reactive microglia are prominent in the perihematomal region on day 1 after ICH, reach a maximum on day 7, and return to normal by 21 days. Similarly, reactive microglia were observed in the perihematomal region as early as1–4 h after whole blood infusion into the rat striatum, peaked at 3–7 days, and persisted for 4 weeks. We have additional data to demonstrate the presence of reactive microglia/macrophages in the perihematomal region 1– 3 days after intrastrial infusion of autologous whole blood. A recent ICH study in rats demonstrated an increase in immunoreactivity of chemokine macrophage inflammatory protein (MIP)-2 that appeared as early as 2 h and peaked at 2 days; the changes in MIP-2 level correlated with nuclear factor-κB activation and brain water content (Wang 2010).

As one type of innate immune cell within the brain, microglia are rapidly activated within 1 h after ICH, peaking at 3–7 days and persisting for several weeks (Yang, Zhong et al. 2015). Microglia are believed to be the first non-neuronal cells to react to brain injury; they act as guardians of neuronal survival and function under various pathologic conditions in the brain. When fully activated, phagocytic microglia are impossible to differentiate from infiltrating macrophages. Increasing evidence suggests that leukocytes/ macrophages, activated microglia, and astrocytes are major cellular mediators of secondary brain damage after ICH based on their local release of cytokines, chemokines, prostaglandins, proteases, ferrous iron, and other immunoactive molecules. Interestingly, cerebral mast cells have gained attention lately, as blocking them has been reported to reduce brain edema and hematoma volume and to improve ICH outcomes (Wang 2010). Hemoglobin is a powerful activator of microglia via toll-like receptors (Wang, Zhou et al. 2014). The imbalance of the phenotypic shift between the M1 and M2 phenotypes of microglia contributes to a large release of ROS in addition to proinflammatory factors (Hu, Tao et al. 2016). Cell experiments have shown that microglia can induce ROS production in vitro. Furthermore, the inhibition of microglia was reported to decrease the ROS production and brain damage volume in an ICH animal model (Hu, Tao et al. 2016).

1.2.2. Astrocytes Reactivation

In the human brain, astrocytes are star-shaped glial cells that generally outnumber neurons by tenfold. Astrocytes are vital for normal brain functions and are considered to be active elements of the brain circuitry. Calcium signaling in activated astrocytes has been proposed to trigger the release of gliotransmitters, such as glutamate, ATP, TNF-α, and d-serine, which can modulate neuronal excitability, synaptic activity, and plasticity. Astrocytes react to many central nervous system injuries and undergo profound morphologic and functional remodeling that is dependent on the type and timing of injury and the distance from the injury site. Disturbance of astrocytic function by brain injury or disease can compromise neuronal functionality and viability. The presence of reactive astrocytes is a hallmark of various neuropathologic conditions. Although astrocytes are recognized to be important in both the initiation and propagation of secondary ischemic brain injury, their contribution to the process of hemorrhagic brain injury has not been clearly defined, and very limited data are available from preclinical or clinical studies (Wang 2010).

Astrocytes, like microglia, are capable of secreting inflammatory mediators. After ICH, brain astrocytes become activated in concert with microglial activation and increase production of glial fibrillary acidic protein (GFAP), causing a so-called "reactive gliosis." Reactive astrogliosis after brain injury could inhibit axonal regeneration. In our two recent studies, we observed a robust activation of astrocytes in the perihematomal region early after ICH that was greatest in regions closest to the injury site and gradually decreased with distance; this pattern was similar to that of microglial activation. Astrocytes were shown to participate in the brain inflammatory process by expressing MMPs after ICH in both the collagenase model and whole-blood model. Interestingly, the presence of blood plasma proteins seems to be an important mediator for activation of astrocytes given that the injection of whole blood induces greater activation of astrocytes than does injection of purified red blood cells. Consistent with the fact that astrocytes have stronger antioxidative potential than do neurons, cultured astrocytes are highly resistant to ROS, and we found that astrocytes are more resistant than neurons to ICH-induced brain injury. The functional significance of the astrocytic response surrounding the hematoma is not totally clear at present. Reactive astrocytes may protect neurons by promoting the secretion of neurotrophic factors or by modulating the expression of microglial inflammatory mediators and microglial ROS production. However, in cases of rapid and severe activation, for example early after ICH, astrocytes are more likely to mediate an inflammatory response to become neurotoxic. Interestingly, reactive astrocytes and microglia can interact to cause local MMP activation. Therefore, controlling microglia–astrocyte interactions could be considered as a potential means to minimize ICH-induced brain injury (Wang 2010). Very few clinical studies have focused on astrocytes after ICH in the human brain. In one early study, researchers investigated brain biopsy specimens from six patients with cerebral amyloid anigiopathy-associated ICH. They found that reactive astrocytes in some patients were labeled with

Alzheimer A4 and gamma-trace peptides, suggesting that astrocytes themselves may have the ability to generate the amyloid peptides (Yong, Robert et al. 1992). In patients with subarachnoid hemorrhage, GFAP concentrations in the cerebrospinal fluid were found to correlate with secondary brain damage caused by delayed cerebral ischemia (Petzold, Keir et al. 2006). One study demonstrated the astrocytic induction of MMP-9 in the perihematomal areas in a postmortem human ICH brain, further supporting the detrimental role of astrocytic overactivation early after ICH (Tejima, Zhao et al. 2007). Thrombin, its endogenous inhibitor protease nexin-1, and water channel protein aquaporin-4 have also been strongly detected by immunohistochemistry in astrocytes, neurons, and cerebral vasculature of the ipsilateral hippocampus at 5–96 h post-ICH in postmortem human brain and experimental ICH (Wu, Zhao et al. 2008, Qing, Dong et al. 2009).

1.2.3. Leukocytes Infiltration

Initially after ICH, leukocytes enter the brain as part of the inflow of blood after vessel rupture. Later, they migrate across the immunologic blood–brain barrier using activated cell adhesion pathways. An important obstacle for a better understanding of the contribution of systemic immune cells to the pathophysiology of ICH is the limitation imposed by the most widely studied experimental models of ICH. Injection of autologous blood allows studying the toxic and immediate inflammatory effects of extravascular blood components, but it fails to reflect the aspect of continuing bleeding. On the contrary, bacterial collagenase dissolves the extracellular matrix around capillaries resulting in active intraparenchymal bleeding because of vessel erosion. However, the vascular source of bleeding in collagenase-induced ICH models differs from most human ICH in which bleeding is of penetrating arterial origin (Mracsko, Javidi et al. 2014).

After ICH induction, some leukocytes are part of the inflowing blood in the hematoma, whereas others actively migrate across the blood–brain barrier. Experimental ICH evokes a similar temporal pattern of cerebral leukocyte infiltration independent of whether autologous blood or collagenase is injected as long as the blood volume is matched. The majority of leukocytes found in the brain after experimental ICH originates from the systemic circulation. CD4+ T lymphocytes are the predominant cerebral leukocyte population in the acute phase of ICH in mice. CD4+ T cells were identified as the predominant subpopulation invading the hemorrhagic brain suggesting a prominent role of T-cell–driven secondary neuroinflammation in ICH. Collagenase injection induces significantly higher numbers of infiltrating granulocytes than blood injection (Mracsko, Javidi et al. 2014).

Preclinical studies of ICH provide substantial histopathologic evidence for the presence of infiltrating leukocytes in and around the hematoma. Neutrophils are the earliest leukocyte subtype to infiltrate into the hemorrhagic brain, and these may damage brain tissue directly by producing ROS, releasing proinflammatory proteases, and modulating BBB permeability. Isolated neutrophils have been shown to aggravate neuronal cell death induced by excitotoxicity or oxygen–glucose deprivation. Once they have entered the hemorrhagic brain, leukocytes will die by apoptosis within two days. The contents of dying leukocytes can further damage brain tissue by stimulating neighboring microglia/macrophages to secrete pro-inflammatory toxic factors. Under a microscope, neutrophils can be identified easily and specifically by using immunohistochemistry with anti-myeloperoxidase antibody. The infiltrating neutrophils appeared in and around the hematoma of mice at 4 h in the collagenase-induced ICH model and that the number of neutrophils peaked at 3 days. This temporal pattern of neutrophil infiltration was reported to be similar in both ICH models in rat (Wang 2010). In patients with ICH, the number of leukocytes present in the cerebrospinal fluid is frequently elevated, and elevated peripheral leukocyte counts have been reported to be positively correlated with hematoma size. In fact, a high peripheral leukocyte count is considered to be an independent predictor of early clinical worsening in primary ICH. To date, three histopathologic studies have examined leukocyte infiltration in the human ICH brain. The first study showed infiltration of neutrophils into the hematoma 2–4 days after ICH. Prior to this infiltration, neutrophil accumulation was observed in blood vessels that bordered the hematoma as early as 6–12 h after ICH. In the second study, investigators examined the early cellular response in postmortem brain tissue and observed that leukocyte infiltration in the peri-ICH region appeared as early as 5–8 h and disappeared by 72 h. The third study examined inflammatory responses and neuronal death in the perihematomal tissue obtained during craniotomy. In that study, infiltration of neutrophils, macrophages, and lymphocytes appeared at 6–12 h and increased further at 12–24 h; the infiltration of these inflammatory cells was correlated with TUNEL-positive cells and expression of Bax protein. Thus, available clinical evidence supports a role for leukocytes in ICH pathogenesis, although the underlying mechanisms involved remain to be determined (Wang 2010).

Monocytes may contribute to secondary injury after intracerebral hemorrhage. There was a positive link between higher admission absolute monocyte count and 30-day case-fatality in ICH (Walsh, Sekar et al. 2015). Recruited leukocytes migrate from the endothelial cell layer by interacting with adhesion molecules on endothelial cells to break through the first mechanical barrier of the BBB (cerebral vascular endothelial cells). Additionally, activated leukocytes can secrete matrix metalloproteinases to activate the plasmin system, and can degrade the extracellular matrix to damage the second mechanical barrier of the BBB (the basement membrane). BBB damage exposes the base of the brain to intravascular serum proteins, moisture, and harmful substances that exosmose and induce vasogenic encephaledema. Encephaledema represents the central link of the secondary attachment of neurons after ICH, and is also a main marker of secondary cerebral injury after ICH (Liu, Shi et al. 2014).

Neutrophils are the leukocyte population that immigrates first into the brain after injury. In ICH, infiltrating neutrophils were found in and around the hematoma as early as 4 h after collagenase-induced ICH in mice. Their number peaks at 3–5 days after ICH. Although the temporal pattern of neutrophil infiltration is similar in blood and collagenase injection models, higher neutrophil numbers are found after collagenase than after blood injection. In experimental ICH, infiltrating neutrophils undergo apoptosis 2 days after entering the hematoma. Molecules released from dying leukocytes may further stimulate microglia/macrophages and exacerbate the neuroinflammatory process. Neutrophil accumulation in the blood vessels around the hematoma was observed already 6 h after the ictus. In the peri-hematomal tissue obtained from ICH patients during craniotomy, neutrophil (and lymphocyte) infiltration further increased 12–24h after ICH and correlated with the number of TUNEL positive cells. It should be noted however that in ischemic stroke histological techniques labeling components of the neurovascular unit showed that polymorphonuclear granulocytes were mainly located in the luminal surfaces or perivascular spaces of cerebral vessels and no granulocytes infiltrated the brain parenchyma. So far, no similar data are available for ICH (Mracsko and Veltkamp 2014).

Recent studies suggest an important role of activated microglia in neutrophil recruitment into the hemorrhagic brain. Heme-induced TLR4 activation on microglia increases CXCL2 production, which interacts with CXCR2 on the surface of neutrophils resulting in chemoattraction. Accordingly, TLR4-deficient mice show reduced neutrophil and monocyte infiltration 3 days after ICH (Mracsko and Veltkamp 2014).

Granulocytes appear to have mainly deleterious effects on the brain after ICH. Neutrophil depletion by intravenous injection of anti-polymorphonuclear neutrophil (anti-PMN) serum reduced BBB breakdown, axonal injury and neurological deficit. After cerebral ischemia, anti-PMN therapy prevented endothelial dysfunction and thrombolysis-induced hemorrhagic transformation in another study. As professional phagocytes, neutrophils use phagosomes containing digestive and oxidative compounds. During phagocytosis they produce an oxidative burst resulting in the release of ROSs via NADPH oxidase and myeloperoxidase. Although these processes are needed for antimicrobial defence, high ROS levels due to microglial activation and neutrophil infiltration contribute to poor outcome after ICH. The free radical scavenger edaravone decreases brain edema and neurological deficit after ICH. Other molecules with free radical trapping properties have been tested in ICH as reviewed earlier supporting the important role of ROS in secondary brain injury and their therapeutic potential after ICH (Mracsko and Veltkamp 2014).

Besides microglia/macrophages, the expression of the neurotoxic TNF-α has also been shown in neutrophils. Neutrophils may also recruit monocyte/macrophages amplifying inflammatory processes. Accordingly, anti-PMN therapy decreased the number of infiltrating monocyte/macrophages around the hematoma and reduced glial scarring (Mracsko and Veltkamp 2014).

Polymorphonuclear neutrophils (PMNs) infiltration into brain parenchyma after cerebrovascular accidents is viewed as a key component of secondary brain injury. The abundance of intraparenchymal PMNs (with no obvious association with vessels) was found in the ICH core and hematoma border, especially between 1 and 7 days after the ictus. The increased presence of intraparenchymal PMNs after ICH coincided with the massive loss of microvascular integrity, suggest vascular disruption as a potential cause of PMNs presence in the brain parenchyma (Liu, Shi et al. 2014).

1.2.4. C-Reactive Protein (CRP)

Although a nonspecific inflammatory marker, the acute phase reactant CRP, has earned popularity in the assessment of inflammation. Yan et al. found significantly higher CRP levels in patients with intracerebral hemorrhage and these levels correlated with worse clinical outcome. Our results also demonstrated higher CRP levels in patients with poor functional outcome and clinical deterioration who were assessed by GOS and MRS. This data gave us substantial evidence to hypothesize that CRP could be a useful marker in predicting ICH prognosis. Significantly higher were found the CRP levels in patients with a history of alcohol abuse. Patients with a history of systemic alcohol abuse demonstrate stronger inflammatory response indicative for worse prognosis (Danovska 2010). Elevation of markers of acute inflammation and hyperglycemia are associated with higher risk of death in patients with sICH, but only CRP is an independent predictor of mortality in these patients (Di Napoli, Godoy et al. 2011).

1.2.5. Cytokines

Cytokines are well-known to be associated with inflammation and immune activation. Although cytokines are released by many cells, including microglia/macrophages, astrocytesand neurons, the major sources of cytokines are activated microglia/macrophages (Wang 2014).

1.2.5.1. TNF-α and IL-1β

Many studies have shown that two major proinflammatory cytokines, TNF-α and interleukin1β (IL-1β), exacerbate ICH-induced brain injury. After ICH, TNF-α is significantly increasedboth *in vivo* and *in vitro*, which may contribute to brain edema formation and braininjury in animal models of ICH. Consistent with animal studies, clinical studies support theproposition that TNF- α contributes to ICH-induced brain injury. Plasma TNF- α has beenshown to correlate with the magnitude of the perihematomal brain edema in patients withICH. Single-nucleotide polymorphisms in the TNF- α gene promoter are associated withspontaneous deep ICH. Similarly, IL-1 β has been found to be upregulated after ICH in ananimal model and to produce detrimental effects, including brain edema and blood - brainbarrier disruption (Wang 2014).

1.2.5.2. Nuclear Factor Kappa-B (NF-κB)

The apoptotic pathway in ICH may involve nuclear factor-kappa B (NF-κB), which is aubiquitous transcription factor that, when activated, translocates to the nucleus and binds toDNA. NF-κB is associated with apoptotic cell death and has been reported in the role of celldeath after experimental ICH in rats. The inflammatory signaling involves a coordinated effort of different molecules and cell typesand is largely coordinated by a ubiquitous transcription factor, NF-κB, a transcription factorinvolved in inflammatory responses, is a key regulator of many proinflammatory cytokines, such as TNF- α , IL-1 β and MMP-9 are involved in various pathological conditions, includingICH-mediated brain injury. Activation of NF-κB occurs within minutes and lasts for at least 1week after the onset of ICH. The activity of NF-κB correlates with perilesional cell death after ICH in rats and is positively associated with the progression of apoptotic cell death in patients with ICH. Several lines of evidence have shown that NF-κB is activated by RBCs and plasmavia signaling pathways involving free radicals, cytokines and glutamate receptors. Cellular necrosis likely occurs at the core of the hemorrhage; however, apoptosis has been observed in the perihematomal region (Wang 2014).

1.2.6. Toll-Like Receptors (TLRs)

Toll-like receptors (TLRs) is expressed in microglia, the resident macrophages of the brain, belong to a large family of pattern recognition receptors that play a key role in innate immunity and inflammatory responses. It has been reported that TLR4 is upregulated in a rat model of ICH and that its signaling pathway contributes to poor outcome after ICH. TLR4 is activated by many endogenous ligands, such as heme and fibrinogen, which are produced in the brain after ICH (Fang, Wang et al. 2013, Wang 2014).

TLR4 is expressed in various cell types in the central nervous system, including microglia, neurons and astrocytes, as well as in peripheral blood cells, such as leukocytes, macrophages and platelets. Microglia are activated within minutes after ICH and subsequently release chemotactic factors to recruit hematogenous phagocytes to the hemorrhagic areas. After ICH, TLR4 mRNA and protein expression is significantly increased by approximately 2 to 6 hours, peaks at day 3, declines somewhat at day 5, but remains elevated relative to baseline even at day 7. Though ICH induces upregulation of TLR4 expression in neurons, astrocytes and microglia, TLR4 is predominantly expressed in CD11b-positive microglial cells in mice. In addition, TLR4 contributes to reduced recruitment of neutrophils and monocytes in the perihematomal area after ICH in TLR4-deficient mice. Therefore, resident microglia in the brain as well as peripheral infiltrating leukocytes and monocytes are likely involved in the roles of TLR4 in ICH-induced brain injury (Fang, Wang et al. 2013).

Exogenous hemin treatment of cultured microglia increases expression of TLR4, as well as proinflammatory cytokines, such as TNF-α, IL-1β and IL-6. This effect is completely abolished by knockout of TLR4 or treatment with anti-TLR4 antibodies, suggesting that TLR4 mediates hemin-stimulated microglial activation. In addition, hemin-induced expression of proinflammatory cytokines TNF-α, IL-1β and IL-6 is completely blocked in TLR4-knockout mice. These data demonstrate that TLR4 signaling mediates heme-induced inflammatory injury, possibly by activating microglial cells and subsequently releasing proinflammatory cytokines. However, Sansing et al.

reported that upregulation of IL-1β and IL-6 genes in the perihematomal region did not significantly differ between TLR4-knockout and WT mice, suggesting that TLR4 signaling may not be involved in the transcriptional regulation of proinflammatory cytokines in perihematomal inflammation. Alternately, it may not be possible to detect upregulation of proinflammatory cytokine genes in certain cell types, such as microglia, when the entire perihematomal region is used (Sansing, Harris et al. 2011, Lin, Yin et al. 2012, Fang, Wang et al. 2013).

Sansing et al. found that TLR4 signaling within the hemorrhage mediated the inflammatory response and contributed to ICH-induced neurological injury. Activation of TLR4 on leukocytes or platelets within the hemorrhage, but not on resident cells, promoted inflammation and resulted in poor functional outcomes. This study clearly demonstrated that TLR4 signaling on peripheral blood cells plays a critical role in ICH-induced brain injury (Sansing, Harris et al. 2011, Lin, Yin et al. 2012, Fang, Wang et al. 2013).

Therefore, TLR4 signaling on resident microglia and on blood cells within the hemorrhage is critical for ICH-induced inflammatory injury. Because TLR4 is expressed on resident microglia which are activated within minutes after ICH, the TLR4 signaling on microglia probably initiates ICH-induced inflammatory injury, causing release of inflammatory cytokines and infiltration of neutrophils. Significant upregulation of TLR4 expression occurs at approximately 2 to 6 hours after ICH, accompanied by the appearance of infiltrating neutrophils in the hematoma (at approximately 4 hours after ICH). TLR4 signaling in the neutrophils may further mediate release of proinflammatory cytokines, which contributes to the detrimental inflammatory response. There are abundant TLR4 activators in the perihematomal region, including heme, fibrinogen and myeloid-related proteins 8 and 14, which are released from degranulating neutrophils. These endogenous activators can stimulate TLR4 on leukocytes, leading to inflammatory injury (Lin, Yin et al. 2012, Fang, Wang et al. 2013).

1.2.7. Complements Activation

Thrombin-induced cerebral injury following ICH may be mediated in large part by complement activation, as inhibition of complement using N-acetylheparin attenuates thrombin-induced edema, complement deposition, and improves neurologic function (Gong, Xi et al. 2005). In the setting of ICH, complement activation results in the rapid induction of multiple parallel downstream pathways of cerebral injury. Cleavage of C3 results in the release of the C3a anaphylatoxin, as well as the association of C3b with C4b2a, producing the C5 convertase. This enzymatic complex cleaves C5, releasing the C5a anaphylatoxin, as well as resulting in the deposition of C5b and subsequent assembly of the pore-forming membrane attack complex (MAC, C5b-9) on the target cell surface. One studyhas proposed a role for complement, specifically for the anaphylatoxin C3a, in neurogenesis following ischemic stroke (Rahpeymai, Hietala et al. 2006). In that study, mice genetically deficient for the C3a receptor, as well as mice treated with an antagonist to the C3a receptor, exhibited impaired basal neurogenesis in the hippocampus. Furthermore, C3 knockout mice exhibited impaired ischemia-induced neurogenesis in the subventri-cular zone following permanent occlusion of the middle cerebral artery. These findings suggest a role for C3a in both basal and ischemia-induced neurogenesis. The role of complement components in neurogenesis following ICH, while a logical extension of this work, remains unexplored. In the setting of ICH, a diffusible anaphylatoxin-mediated response, as well as MAC-mediated lysis of erythrocytes, subserve distinct but parallel roles in exacerbating perihematomal cerebral injury. The anaphylatoxins C3a and C5a serve as powerful chemoat-tractants for leukocytes and may damage the blood–brain barrier following ICH. Anaphylatoxin induction induces rapid activation of endothelial cells and resident microglia, as well as infiltration of granulocytes, in the perihematomal region (Rynkowski, Kim et al. 2008). Activated microglia secrete inflammatory cytokines such as TNF-α and IL-1β, thereby amplifying the inflammatory response (Aronowski and Hall 2005). Inflammatory cells also release myeloperoxidase and other toxic products when activated, producing reactive oxygen species which cause direct cerebral injury. These coordinated responses culminate in an exacerbation of brain edema, leading to secondary cerebral injury (Xi, Hua et al. 2002, Rynkowski, Kim et al. 2009). The formation of the MAC promotes erythrocyte lysis is a parallel injury pathway following ICH. This pathway enhances brain edema in both the acute and delayed phases and functions through a mechanism relying on the breakdown of hemoglobin, which is degraded by heme oxygenase into iron, carbon monoxide, and biliverdin (Wu, Hua et al. 2003). Hua and colleagues provided the first direct evidence for complement activation in ICH and its involvement in cerebral edema formation (Hua, Xi et al. 2000). Increased perihematomal C9 was detected 24 h following the injection of autologous blood into rat basal ganglia and MAC formation was evident by 72 h. Evidence also suggests that MAC may be directly injurious to neurons, astrocytes, and endothelial cells leading to blood–brain barrier disruption (Bellander, Singhrao et al. 2001).

1.2.8. Matrix Metalloproteinases

Matrix metalloproteinases (MMPs) are a large family of zinc-dependent endopeptidases involved in extracellular remodeling as well as the neuroinflammatory response. To date, 23 MMPs have been identified in humans (Gueders, Foidart et al. 2006). MMPs are normally located in the cytosol in a pro- or inactivated state; however, under pathologic conditions, they are cleaved by proteases, such as plasmin, tissue plasminogen activator (tPA), or other MMPs, to their active state. Accordingly, expression of MMPs in the normal brain is very low, but many MMPs are upregulated and activated in response to various brain injuries (Xue, Fan et al. 2009).

Preclinical studies of MMPs in ICH have focused on MMP-2, -3, -9, and -12. The first such study, by Rosenberg and Navratil, demonstrated that gelatinases MMP-2 and MMP-9 were activated within 24 h of collagenase-induced ICH in rats. Other investigators observed increases in mRNA levels of MMP-3 and/or -12 (Wells, Biernaskie et al. 2005). Early increases in MMP-9 mRNA, protein, and/or activity have been confirmed in other ICH studies that have used different animal models. Recently, Xue and colleaguesobserved that human recombinant MMP-3 and -9 can directly kill human fetal neurons. In support of this finding, mice with genetic deletions for MMP-3, -9, and -12 were reported to have less hemorrhagic brain injury than wild-type (WT) mice after ICH, although contrary results for MMP-9 were reported in one study. Furthermore, MMP-3 and -9 were reported to act synergistically with thrombin (Wang 2010).

Several clinical studies have reported that blood MMP-9 levels are increased in patients with acute spontaneous ICH. This increase in blood MMP-9 levels within 12 or 24 h after stroke onset is associated with subsequent enlargement of the hematoma, perihematomal edema, and worsening of neurologic function. Alvarez-Sabin et al. (2004) systematically investigated the temporal profile of MMPs and their natural inhibitors in patients with acute ICH and found that an increase in blood MMP-9 levels correlated with perihematomal edema and neurologic deterioration during the acute stage, whereas elevated blood MMP-3 levels were associated with mortality. Moreover, increasing evidence identifies an association between elevated MMP-9 concentration and subsequent hemorrhagic transformation or thrombolytic-induced hemorrhage in ischemic stroke patients. In one recent study, investigators observed an association between plasma levels of MMP-9 and BBB disruption after stroke in humans. To date, only two histopathologic studies have been identified in which MMPs were examined in human ICH brain within the first 6 h after death. The results showed that MMP-9 was upregulated in neurons and reactive astrocytes surrounding the hematoma; brain tissue around the hemotoma had higher MMP-9 levels than did the contralateral hemisphere, supporting a contribution of MMP-9 to perihematomal edema. Taken together, available clinical data support detrimental roles for MMP-9 in ICH and hemorrhagic transformation after ischemic stroke; however, the roles of MMP-3 and -12 still need to be studied in clinical settings (Wang 2010).

1.3. Hemolysis Products

1.3.1. Hemoglobin

Hemoglobin (Hb) is a major component of blood and a potent mediator of oxidative stress after ICH (Katsu, Niizuma et al. 2010). As the most abundant erythrocyte protein, hemoglobin is released into the extracellular space via complement-mediated cell lysis in the hours after ICH and is a potent mediator of OS-induced injury. Hemoglobin released from extravasated erythrocytes is implicated in brain edema after ICH. Hemoglobin is a major component of blood and a potent mediator of oxidative stress after ICH (Wang, Yang et al. 2011). Hemoglobin and its degradation products, heme and iron, are potent cytotoxic components that can induce cell death and disrupt the blood –brain-barrier. The prominent mechanism of Hb toxicity is via the generation of free radicals (mainly through a Fenton-type mechanism) and the resulting oxidative damage to proteins, nucleic acids, carbohydrates, and lipids (Wang, Manaenko et al. 2016). Our study also showed that hemoglobin levels reached a plateau at 3 days after ICH, and which triggered the scavenging pathway to remove it (Wang, Manaenko et al. 2016). Both in vitro and in vivo investigations have shown that ROS is highly produced after exposing Hb to cell culture or injecting Hb into mouse striatum. Katsu et al. studied the temporal change of ROS in a Hb-injection rat model and observed remarkable ROS production as early as 1 h, which increased at 24 h. Recently, NO, a form of RNS, has also been found to be overproduced because of NOS activation and leads to BBB disruption after infusing Hb into rat brain. Regarding the prooxidant mechanism of Hb, it is commonly believed that iron released from its degradation is responsible for oxidative damage because an iron chelator may block Hb-induced neurotoxicity. In fact, Hb itself can release a large amount of superoxide during spontaneous, nonenzymatic oxidation to oxyhemoglobin and methemoglobin (Hu, Tao et al. 2016). Hb-induced oxidative stress may contribute to early BBB dysfunction and subsequent apoptosis, partly through

MMP activation, and that SOD1 overexpression may reduce Hb-induced oxidative stress, BBB dysfunction, and apoptotic cell death (Katsu, Niizuma et al. 2010). Hemoglobin (Hb), heme, and iron released after red blood cell lysis aggravate ICH-induced inflammatory injury.

1.3.2. Heme

Free heme does not accumulate normally in tissue; it is deposited in tissues only under pathologic conditions. The term 'free heme' is used in reference to the molecule before its incorporation into hemoproteins. The molecule is integral to life as part of hemoproteins; and as such, carries out oxidative reactions, electron transfer processes, and delivers molecular oxygen (O2) to cells (Chang, Claus et al. 2005). Heme is a major component of hemoproteins, released from methemoglobin, quickly oxidizes to form hemin, which also triggers oxidative damage in brain tissue around the hematoma. Free heme is deposited in tissue only in pathological conditions. Hemorrhage, ischemia, edema, and mechanical injury damage are all processes that may result in the release of heme from hemoproteins (Chang, Claus et al. 2005). Intracellular heme originates from cytoplasmic hemoproteins and from mitochondrial cytochromes located in neurons and glia (Wagner, Sharp et al. 2003). Extracellular heme is released from dying cells and from extravasated hemoglobin from red blood cells [9]. The release of oxyhemoglobin (oxyHb) leads to superoxide anion (02•) and hydrogen peroxide (H202) release as oxyhemoglobin undergoes auto-oxidation to methemeglobin. Free heme is degraded by heme oxygenase-1 (HO-1) and heme oxygenase-2 (HO-2) into Fe2+, CO, and one isomer of biliverdin, which rapidly reduces to free bilirubin. Free heme is lipophilic and enhances lipid peroxidation. An in vitro experiment demonstrated that hemin exposure leads to cell death, preceded by a significant, iron-dependent increase in ROS. Nevertheless, another in vitro study showed that hemin could stimulate lipid peroxidation, irrespective of iron mediation, because the reaction could not be inhibited by deferoxamine or transferrin. Hence, the mechanism of hemin-related oxidative damage partly involves its breakdown to iron by HO, similar to that of Hb. Indeed, hemin is redox-active and can react with peroxides to produce cytotoxic free radicals. Moreover, hemin can intercalate into the cell plasma membrane, facilitating lipid peroxidation. Given the effect of hemin in preclinical studies, biphasic functions are observed. Hemin-induced brain injury is evidenced by increased brain water content at 24 hours after intracerebral hemin infusion. In contrast, systemic hemin treatment is neuroprotective after ICH. Although the mechanisms underlying the protection provided by systemic hemin administration are poorly understood, it is clear that most hemin is in circulation rather than in the brain (Hu, Tao et al. 2016). Cytoplasmic hemoproteins and mitochondrial cytochromes in neurons and glia are intracellular sources of heme. Extracellular sources of heme include hemoproteins that are released from dying cells, and/or derived from hemoglobin that is generated as a consequence of subarachnoid and intraparenchymal bleeding. Extravascular erythrocytes lyse in the central nervous system (CNS) via a complement-mediated mechanism. Furthermore, extracellular hemoglobin is thought to be selectively internalized by microglia throughout the brain after experimental subarachnoid hemorrhage, possibly mediated through the induction of hemopexin. Heme and the products of heme catabolism have all been shown to be distinct bioactive molecules and therefore the subject of considerable interest (Chang, Claus et al. 2005). Heme is degraded by heme oxygenases (HOs) into biliverdin, iron, and carbon monoxide, and heme itself or its degradation products may contribute to formation of brain edema.

1.3.3. Iron

Iron overload is involved in secondary brain injury, leading to neuronal death, brain edema, and neurodeficits after ICH. Iron, a major hemoglobin degradation product which accumulates in the brain parenchyma for months, has a detrimental effect in secondary injury. Iron plays a key role in edema formation and cell death after ICH. Prominently, the mechanism of iron toxicity includes generating free radicals (mainly through Fenton-type mechanism) and directly compromising the neighboring brain cells. Reactive oxygen species (ROS) can directly or indirectly damage all biomolecules, including proteins, lipids, deoxyribonucleic acid (DNA), and carbohydrates Intracerebral iron overload begins within 24 h, peaks at 7 days, and continues for at least a month after hemorrhage (Wang, Hu et al. 2015). Excessive iron in the extracellular space induces oxidative damage via the Fenton reaction, which yields ROS, especially toxic hydroxyl radicals. Direct evidence of iron-mediated oxidative injury has shown that injecting FeCl2 into rat brain causes oxidative DNA damage. The strongest finding supporting the hypothesis of iron-mediated oxidative brain injury is that iron chelators decrease iron accumulation, attenuate ROS generation, exert anti-inflammatory effects, and improve neurological function (Hu, Tao et al. 2016). Excess ferrous iron is deemed to be a major source of oxidative stress due to the production of reactive oxygen species (ROS) through Fenton reaction. The reaction involves the process of inducing the ferrous iron and hydrogen peroxide into a toxic hydroxide ion and a hydroxyl free radical, with the concurrent oxidation of ferrous iron to ferric iron. The ability of the ferrous iron to generate ROS and hydroxyl radicals initiates lipid peroxidation as well as direct DNA damage (Wang, Shao et al. 2015). Our study results demonstrated that iron overload (especially ferrous iron) plays a key role in brain secondary injury after ICH (Qing, Dong et al. 2009, Wang, Hu et al. 2015, Wang, Shao et al. 2015). So ferrous iron may be a promising target for ICH in future.

1.3.4. Heme Oxygenase

Heme is degraded by heme oxygenase (HO) into three highly bioactive products: iron, bilirubin, and carbon monoxide. The HO isozymes, in particular HO-1 and HO-2, exhibit significantly different expression patterns and appear to have specific roles after injury. Extracellular heme binds to hemopexin to enter neuronal cells through the hemopexin receptor or heme carrier protein 1. Intracellular heme is then degraded into iron, carbon monoxide, and biliverdin. HO is the rate-limiting enzyme for this catabolic process with two active isoenzymes: the inducible HO-1 and the constitutively active HO-2. HO-1 is barely detected in the brain under normal conditions but is induced in microglia/macrophages after ICH, whereas HO-2 is normally expressed in neurons, accounting for the vast majority of HO activity in the brain (Munoz-Sanchez and Chanez-Cardenas 2014).

The antioxidant effects of these enzymes on ICH-induced secondary brain injury are debatable and have been thoroughly reviewed by Chen-Roetling et al. Their roles are variable, depending on the different ICH models used and various cellular types affected (Chen-Roetling, Lu et al. 2015). Compared to wild-type mice, HO-2 knockout was found to attenuate brain injury, remarkably reducing cell loss, striatal protein, and lipid oxidation in a blood-injection model, but worsened the outcome by increasing perihematomal lesion volume, neuroinflammation, and edema in a collagenase-injection model (Chen-Roetling, Cai et al. 2014). Conversely, HO-1 knockout exerted a beneficial effect on outcome in a collagenase-induced ICH model (Wang and Dore 2007). These disparate conclusions are partly explained by the diverse injury mechanisms between the blood- and collagenase-injection ICH models and the different distributions and expression timing of HO-1 and HO-2 (Chen-Roetling, Lu et al. 2015, Hu, Tao et al. 2016).

Because of the potential harmful effects of hemoglobin (Hb) breakdown, HO-1 and HO-2 activity may be detrimental after TBI. However, HO-1 increased heme catabolism, the product of carbon monoxide and biliverdin, so it plays a protective role against oxidative injuries in the vascular system.

There is also evidence that HO-1 is neuroprotective (Wang, Yang et al. 2011). But contradictory results have been found in twoclinical trials, bilirubin (known to be a powerful antioxidant), HO-1 and peroxidized lipid content were significantly higher in cerebrospinal fluid (CSF) from subarachnoid hemorrhage (SAH) patients with vasospasm, compared with nonvasospasm SAH CSF, and correlated with occurrence of vasospasm. It is suggested that bilirubin and HO-1was induced after hemorrhagic stroke, reflecting the intensity of oxidative stress. Moreover HO-1 leads to iron accumulation, iron-induced oxidation causes DNA damage in brain after ICH and that iron is a therapeutic target for ICH. Oxidative stress plays an important role and contributes to the pathophysiology of ICH (Katsu, Niizuma et al. 2010). HO-1, as a major rate-limiting enzyme of iron production and heme reduction, its role in the pathogenesis of ICH is controversial. Our research results showed that HO-1 may play a protective role as an antioxidant at early stage following ICH. Whereas it may be a prooxidant at late stage post-ICH. Its early mild upregulation possibly is adaptive response to brain acute insult, whereas the overexpression of HO-1 in the latter stages possibly exacerbate or reflect oxidative status. It suggested that HO-1 has both antioxidant and prooxidant properties in ICH. Upregulation of HO-1 after ICH may be a double-edged sword. The early mild upregulation possibly fit with the events and its overexpression in the late stages may result in its dysfunction and be toxic. It should be prudent to intervene ICH with the inhibitor or activator of HO-1 and think over its potential dual effects (Wang, Yang et al. 2011). It happened to coincide with the aforementioned contradictory results of clinical trials.

1.3.5. Bilirubin

Intracerebral infusion of bilirubin caused an increase in brain water content at 24 hours (Huang, Xi et al. 2002). Following ICH, amounts of unconjugated bilirubin in hematoma can be substantial, as can levels of iron and hemoglobin. Oxidation of unconjugated bilirubin to yield bioactive molecules, such as production of bilirubin oxidation products (BOXes) expanding the role of bilirubin in pathological processes seen after ICH (Clark, Loftspring et al. 2008). Unconjugated bilirubin (UBR) increases inflammatory cell infiltration and edema after ICH (Loftspring, Johnson et al. 2011). With regard to neutrophil function, it seems that low UBR has proinflammatory properties, whereas high UBR suppresses certain functions. For example, in vitro high UBR (45 μmol/L) suppressed superoxide production. In vivo, UBR was associated with decreased nitrate/nitrite. This could occur either by direct scavenging of reactive oxygen species or by altering signaling pathways (Datla,

Dusting et al. 2007). Datla et al. (2007) observed a concentration-dependent inhibition of superoxide production by UBR in HL-60 cells (Datla, Dusting et al. 2007). UBR may induce degranulation of neutrophil collagenases in vivo leading to increased brain edema. This is plausible because higher UBR was required for degranulation than for potentiation of superoxide production in vitro. This possibility is in accordance with our finding of increased PKC+ neutrophils in the UBR group. Unconjugated bilirubin has previously been shown to cause edema in experimental ICH (Huang, Xi et al. 2002). Gordo et al. (2006) have shown that UBR activates and then damages the microglia in vitro, causing them to become necrotic (Gordo, Falcao et al. 2006). Unconjugated bilirubin activates specific signaling pathways in the microglia as opposed to only causing generalized toxicity. Silva et al. (2010) have recently found in vitro that UBR is associated with mitogen-activated protein kinase and nuclear factor-κB activation within 2 hours of UBR exposure (Silva, Vaz et al. 2010). Therefore, UBR in ICH may be associated with hyperacute microglia activation followed by later cell death. These results are significant because they suggest that the concentration of UBR and cell type (s) on which it acts are important determinants of whether it is proinflammatory or anti-inflammatory (Loftspring, Johnson et al. 2011).

1.4. Oxidative Stress

Oxidative stress basically defines a condition in which prooxidant-antioxidant balance in the cell is disturbed; cellular biomolecules undergo severe oxidative damage, ultimately compromising cells viability. In recent years, a number of studies have shown that oxidative stress could cause cellular apoptosis via both the mitochondria-dependent and mitochondria-independent pathways. Oxidative stress is a condition in which the overproduction of free radicals, mainly reactive oxygen species (ROS), exceeds the antioxidant capacity and subsequently leads to cell injury via directly oxidizing cellular protein, lipid, and DNA or participating in cell death signaling pathways (Sinha, Das et al. 2013). Oxidative stress has been implicated in neurodegenerative diseases of the central nervous system and stroke (Manzanero, Santro et al. 2013). There are three major types of ROS: the superoxide radical (O2·−), the hydroxyl radical (OH), and hydrogen peroxide (H2O2) (Mates, Segura et al. 2012). Reactive nitrogen species (RNS) are another major type of free radicals, which mainly consist of nitric oxide (NO) and its derivatives. NO is produced in neurons, endothelial cells, and activated astrocytes by nitric oxide synthase (NOS). Under physiological conditions, NO mediates neurotransmission and regulates neuronal survival, proliferation, and differentiation. Under pathological conditions, however, excessive NO can lead to OS via various mechanisms. Moreover, NO reacts with $O2^{\cdot-}$ to form the more toxic compound peroxynitrite ($ONOO^{-}$), which can cause oxidation and nitration of tyrosine residues in proteins (Ding, Chen et al. 2014, Hu, Tao et al. 2016). Moreover, Increased leukocyte8-hydroxy-2′ -deoxyguanosine (8-OHdG) levels, as well as decreased erythrocyte glutathione peroxidase (GPx) activity and vitamin E levels, were found during acute ICH. Only 8-OHdG was associated with ICH and the 30-day outcome independently from the other oxidative markers and traditional factors. Leukocyte 8-OHdG may add power beyond the traditional factors in predicting ICH outcome and thus may be used as an independent surrogate for clinical ICH study (Chen, Chen et al. 2011). The other oxidative markers, serum C-reactive protein (CRP) and lipid hydroperoxides (ROOH) were predictors of short-term mortality after after spontaneous ICH. Although serum ROOH level was positively correlated with mortality, it did not predict early lethal outcome. Serum ROOH concentration, however, was a predictor of poor clinical outcome in sICH survivors. After confirmation of the results obtained through observing a larger group of patients, an oxidative stress marker could be used as an additional criterion for patient stratification, especially when severe disability is expected and supplementary therapeutic approaches are urgent (Alexandrova and Danovska 2011).

2. Therapeutic Options to Attenuate Secondary Injury Following ICH

2.1. Surgery Approach

Because intraparenchymal blood is the origin of many prooxidant toxins, including Hb, heme, and iron, it is reasonable to suppose that blood evacuation may reduce oxidative damage if the surgery results in no or minimal additional new injury. Hence, minimally invasive surgery (MIS) for clot evacuation may represent a therapeutic strategy for the prevention of secondary oxidative damage. Animal studies have demonstrated that MIS alone or combined with other therapy can improve neurofunction with decreased oxidative injury and reduced apoptosis (Liu, Jing et al. 2016). More recently, clinical trials with small sample sizes investigating newly applied mechanical devices have reported promising outcomes (Przybylowski, Ding et al. 2015). A multicenter, randomized, controlled study comparing MIS with routine craniotomy is ongoing and involves 2448 ICH patients (Zielinski, Jongsma et al. 2014). The clinical results will provide valuable information regarding the effect of MIS on the prognosis of patients with ICH (Hu, Tao et al. 2016). Clinical trials evaluating the surgical removal of hematomas have not achieved the expected results (Mendelow, Gregson et al. 2013).

So there are some recommendations for surgical treatment of ICH (showed in Table1-3):

1. Patients with cerebellar hemorrhage who are deteriorating neurologically or who have brainstem compression and/or hydrocephalus from ventricular obstruction should undergo surgical removal of the hemorrhage as soon as possible (Class I; Level of Evidence B). Initial treatment of these patients with ventricular drainage rather than surgical evacuation is not recommended (Class III; Level of Evidence C). (Unchanged from the previous guideline)
2. For most patients with supratentorial ICH, the usefulness of surgery is not well established (Class IIb; Level of Evidence A).
3. A policy of early hematoma evacuation is not clearly beneficial compared with hematoma evacuation when patients deteriorate (Class IIb; Level of Evidence A). (New recommendation)
4. Supratentorial hematoma evacuation in deteriorating patients might be considered as a life-saving measure (Class IIb; Level of Evidence C). (New recommendation)
5. DC with or without hematoma evacuation might reduce mortality for patients with supratentorial ICH who are in a coma, have large hematomas with significant midline shift, or have elevated ICP refractory to medical management (Class IIb; Level of Evidence C). (New recommendation)
6. The effectiveness of minimally invasive clot evacuation with stereotactic or endoscopic aspiration with or without thrombolytic usage is uncertain (Class IIb; Level of Evidence B) (Hemphill, Greenberg et al. 2015).

2.2. Potential Nonsurgery Approach

2.2.1. Thrombin Intervention

Hirudin-a thrombin inhibitor/ deactivator, was administered at 5 min (early) after ICH, microglia activation and leukocyte infiltration were significantly inhibited, while CD34-positivemicrovessel abundance could be restored to normal levels, indicating that thrombin-induced BBB damage was reversible and early hirudin application could minimize BBB damage. When hirudin was applied 24 h after ICH (the edematization stage), hirudin could still inhibit microglia activation and leukocyte infiltration, but it did not significantly increase the number of CD34-positive microvessels. These findings suggest that hirudin can inhibit perihematomal in flammatory reactions, but it cannot reverse BBB damage, indicating that the inhibition of hirudin on vasogenic encephaledema has a specific mechanism of action and is most effective when administered quickly. Specifically, the intervention treatment must be conducted in the early stages of activation of these cells and a positive outcome can be achieved only when tissues are in a reversible stage of injury. If the damage exceeds the thresholds of cells, it will cause irreversible cell death. This study provides a theoretical basis for the early application ofanti-thrombin drugs to block thrombin-mediated toxicity after ICH in clinical settings (Liu, Shi et al. 2014).

2.2.2. Inflammation Intervention

2.2.2.1. Upstream Inflammatory Signal Inhibition

Excessive inflammatory responses, both central and peripheral inflammation, contribute to secondary brain injury following ICH, while modest inflammation promotes the neurogenesis. At present most studies concentrated on the downstream inflammatory events, such as proinflammatory cytokines, showed that inflammatory responses contribute to the secondary brain injury after ICH, while no direct clinical effects on targeting these downstream events have been achieved. So it's necessary to explore the upstream events that initiate the inflammatory cascade after ICH. Recently, one study showed that microglia toll-like receptor 4 (TLR4) triggers the upstream inflammatory signal to cause secondary brain injury, which was attenuated by TLR4 antagonist TAK242. Subsequently, they found a novel TLR2/ TLR4 heterodimer triggered by Hb that initiates the excessive inflammatory responses following ICH, and intervening the TLR2/TLR4 heterodimer with sparstolonin B (SsnB), a Chinese herb-derived compound, has also achieved markedly antiinflammatory effects and improved the neurologic deficit following ICH (Xiong and Yang 2015). SsnB, as a Chinese herb monomer, can not only inhibit the central but also the peripheral TLRs signaling to reduce the upstream inflammatory events that caused brain injury; meanwhile, it would not change the blood immune cell quantities which avoid increasing infection risk. So, it may have a better application prospect for the ICH treatment. However, further study should perform to investigate the clinical effects of SsnB in the ICH patients, in particular, targeting the inflammatory cascade in the early stage to reduce secondary brain injury and keeping a modest inflammation milieu in the late stage to promote neurogenesis and recovery. Therefore, seeking an appropriate treatment time window for the ICH treatment and targeting the upstream events of inflammation may provide a better therapeutic strategy (Xiong and Yang 2015).

A specific antibody (Mts50) blocked TLR4 signaling in a mouse model of ICH. TLR4 antibody treatment significantly reduced cerebral water content and improved neurological function after ICH, similar to effects observed in TLR4-knockout mice, suggesting that blockade of the TLR4 receptor is a potential therapeutic approach in the treatment of ICH (Fang, Wang et al. 2013). The neuroprotective effects of the TLR4 antibody in ICH may be associated with inhibition of cytokine expression and macrophage infiltration. However, the effectiveness of the antibody on hemin-induced TLR4 activation in macrophages is controversial. One study found that the TLR4 antibody effectively suppressed hemin-induced microglial activation in mice. However, Figueiredo et al. reported that this antibody blocked only LPS-induced, but not hemin-induced, TLR4 activation in macrophages, suggesting that different TLR4 receptor conformations exist in response to different ligands. The discrepancy between the two studies may be due to use of different reagents and animal models, and further studies are needed to evaluate the efficacy of the TLR4 antibody for ICH (Fang, Wang et al. 2013).

Many TLR4 antagonists have been reported to produce anti-inflammatory effects. Some antagonists, such as curumin, 6-shogaol, isoliquiritigenin, and OSL07 (4-oxo-4- (2-oxo-oxazolidin-3-yl)-but-2-enoic acid ethyl ester), block TLR4 signaling by inhibiting homodimerization of TLR4. Other agents, such as sparstolonin B, auranofin, TAK-242, and M62812, have also been reported to block TLR4 signaling pathways selectively. However, most of these agents were tested in an animal model of LPS-induced sepsis. The effects of these agents on ICH-induced inflammation have not yet been explored (Fang, Wang et al. 2013).

In addition to these antagonists, many agents with multiple pharmacological mechanisms have been found to have neuroprotective effects in animal models of ICH via inhibition of TLR4 signaling. For example, oxymatrine, which has anti-inflammatory, antioxidative, and antiapoptotic activities, suppresses TLR4 and NF-κB gene expression and decreases production of proinflammatory cytokines, such as IL-6, TNF-α, and IL-1β. Ginkgolide B, a specific platelet-activating factor receptor antagonist, reduces neuronal cell apoptosis after traumatic brain injury in rats, possibly via inhibition of TLR4 signaling pathways. Progesterone treatment inhibits TLR4 signaling pathways and reduces brain edema and blood–brain barrier impairment after subarachnoid hemorrhage in rats. These agents are not specific TLR4 receptor blockers, but they can inhibit TLR4 signaling to reduce ICH-induced inflammatory injury. It has been reported that progesterone inhibits TLR4/NF-κB signaling pathway and decrease proinflammatory cytokine production in rats following subarachnoid hemorrhage, suggesting that suppressed proinflammatory signaling may contribute to preconditioning by TLR4 activation in ICH. Therefore, suppressed proinflammatory signaling and/or enhanced anti-inflammatory IFN signaling may be associated with preconditioning by TLR4 activation in ICH (Fang, Wang et al. 2013). Additional studies of the mechanisms of preconditioning by TLR4 activation in ICH are warranted.

2.2.2.2. Anti- Inflammatory Agents

Urocortin (UCN), a novel anti-inflammatory neuropeptide, protects injured cardiomyocytes and dopaminergic neurons. One study indicates UCN alleviates ICH-induced brain injury when administered intracerebroventricularly (ICV). Systemic post-ICH treatment with UCN reduces striatal injury and neurological deficits, likely via suppression of microglial activation and inflammatory cytokine production. The low dose of UCN necessary and the clinically amenable peripheral route make UCN a potential candidate for development into a clinical treatment regimen. However, the biological activities of UCN in inflammation remain controversial. Although most studies agree that UCN is a powerful anti-inflammatory agent, some have found a pro-inflammatory effect, causing vasculitis and increased pulmonary vascular permeability. This disparity may be due to the different subtypes of CRF receptors distributed in the CNS and periphery, and different cells and tissues, or to different effects of UCN in local and systemic administration (Liew, Pang et al. 2012).

Anti-inflammatory therapies have been tested in preclinical and clinical studies, but the efficacy of anti-inflammatory agents have not been documented in clinical use so far. Therapeutic hypothermia has been extensively studied as a means to reduce ischemic or hemorrhagic brain injury through its anti-inflammatory effect. Although therapeutic hypothermia provides considerable protection after ischemic stroke, evidence for a beneficial effect in ICH is insufficient, and potential complications can arise, such as infection and increased blood pressure. Thus, its clinical usefulness for ICH is in question (Wang 2010).

2.2.2.3. Microglia Inhibition

Therapeutic strategies based on the inhibition of microglial activation have been tested in preclinical trials. In two of early studies, authors pretreated (2 days before) or post-treated (2 h after) mice with MIF (microglia/macrophage inhibitory factor, tuftsin fragment 1–3, Thr-Lys-Pro) to inhibit microglial activation. MIF-treated mice showed reduced brain injury and improved neurologic function. Similarly, inhibition of microglial activation with minocycline, which also inhibits MMPs, was shown to protect the BBB, reduce brain edema, and thereby improve functional recovery in collagenase-induced ICH in rats, although neuronal loss was not decreased. Neuroprotection conferred by minocycline also was reported in rodents subjected to the whole-blood model and will be discussed in depth below. However, negative results have also been reported. Although cumulatively the data suggest that strategies to target early inhibition of microglia/macrophage activation after ICH could be therapeutic, long-term inhibition may not be fully beneficial because inhibition could potentially abolish neuroprotective benefits of microglia/macrophages as phagocytes and suppliers of neuroreactive molecules (Wang 2010).

One way to control neuroinflammation is to inhibit microglial activation. Studies on microglia have shown that they are activated by diverse stimuli but they are dependent on activation of mitogen-activated protein kinase (MAPK). Previous approaches to down-regulate activated microglia focused on immunosuppressants. Recently, minocycline (a tetracycline derivative) has shown down-regulation of microglial MAPK. Another promising treatment is CPI-1189, which induces cell death in a tumor necrosis factor (TNF) α - inhibiting compound that also down-regulates MAPK. Recent study shows that nicergoline (Sermion) suppresses the production of proinflammatory cytokines and superoxide anion by activated microglia. Microglial activation can be inhibited by MIF (microglia/macrophage inhibitory factor, tufts infragment 1 - 3, Thr-Lys-Pro). MIF-treated mice showed reduced brain injury and improved neurologic function in a mouse model of collagenase-induced intracerebral hemorrhage. Albeit some inflammatory responses generated by microglia/macrophages after ICH may aggravate brain injury, microglia/macrophages-mediated phagocytosis is instrumental in conducting brain clean-up, the process that must occur to allow for tissue repair and functional recovery. A fast and efficient removal of apoptotic, dislocated (e.g., extravascular erythrocytes), and damaged cells before the discharge of injurious and proinflammatory cell contents (damage associated molecular patterns) occurs and may help to reduce secondary damage. So, by inhibiting the activation of microglial cells, namely the inhibition of brain primary response to the timely removal of damaged tissue and self repairing systems, to reduce the amount of potential damages, the desirability of this way is still questionable (Wang 2014).

Hyperbaric oxygen preconditioning (HBOP) could significantly alleviate the ICH-induced neuroinflammation by regulating microglia characteristics changing (Yang, Tang et al. 2015).

2.2.2.4. Reduction in Leucocyte Infiltration

Fingolimod, a sphingosine 1-phosphate receptor analog, prevents the egress of lymphocytes from primary and secondary lymphoid organs. Fingolimod treatment ameliorated cerebral inflammation, at least to some extent, by reducing the availability and subsequent brain infiltration of T-lymphocytes, which improved the short and long-term sequelae after experimental ICH in rodents (Rolland, Lekic et al. 2013). HO-1−/− mice are significantly protected from early brain injury and functional impairment produced by ICH. This protection appeared to be associated with a reduction in leucocyte infiltration, microglia/macrophage activation and ROS production during the critical phase of the early post-ICH period (Wang and Dore 2007).

2.2.2.5. Metalloproteinases Inhibitor

Given the proposed detrimental effect of metalloproteinases (MMPs) activity early after ICH, several investigators have used inhibitors to block MMP activity in preclinical studies. Rosenberg and Navratil reported that rats treated with BB-1101 (a broad-spectrum hydroxamic acid-based MMP inhibitor) reduced brain edema and mortality when administrated 6 h after the onset of ICH. Treatment of mice with the broad-spectrum MMP inhibitor GM6001 attenuated gelatinase activity, neutrophil infiltration, and ROS production, and thereby decreased early brain injury and improved neurologic function. Neuroprotection conferred by GM6001 was further confirmed in a mouse study that used the whole-blood model of ICH. Two early studies reported that MMP inhibition with BB-94 reduced recombinant tPA-induced hemorrhage after thromboembolic stroke and recombinant tPA-related mortality after middle cerebral artery occlusion. In contrast, Grossetete and Rosenberg reported that MMP inhibition with BB-94 increased cell death and hemorrhage volume in a collagenase-induced ICH mouse model (Wang 2010).

Minocycline, a semi-synthetic tetracycline, has shown promise as a MMP inhibitor and a neuroprotectant. Power et al. (2003) reported that inhibition of MMP-12 with minocycline protected the morphology of neurons and improved functional recovery after ICH. Although delayed administration of minocycline (6 h post-ICH) failed to reduce neuronal death or striatal tissue loss at day 7, it did decrease early upregulation of TNF-α and MMP-12, thereby protecting the BBB and reducing brain edema. Contrary to these positive results, one study reported that minocycline provided neither histologic nor functional protection when administrated 3 h after ICH, even though the number of microglia/macrophages was reduced in the perihematomal areas. Together, most of the preclinical findings support the view that MMP-3, -9, and -12 might play a detrimental role in the pathophysiology of ICH and that intervention with MMP inhibitors might decrease ICH-induced early brain injury. However, the timing of MMP inhibition is critical, and long-term inhibition can be deleterious because MMPs do exert beneficial effects during neurovascular remodeling and recovery in the later phases of ICH (Wang 2010).

2.2.2.6. Complement Cascade Intervention

A multitude of pharmacologic strategies exist for targeting the complement cascade as a therapeutic intervention in a particular disease process. Given the redundancy of the proximal pathways of activation, the possibility for cascade-independent cleavage of C3, and available evidence derived from experimental models, strategies targeting C3 are currently the most attractive choice for complement inhibition following ICH. This strategy would serve to inhibit the formation of both anaphylatoxins, as well as the downstream process of MAC-mediated erythrocyte lysis, and concomitant heme toxicity. However, given the known role for complement in the clearance of apoptotic cell bodies, as well as its putative role in ICH-induced neurogenesis, therapeutic complement inhibition must be carried out in a temporally targeted fashion to maximize the beneficial effects of complement inhibition while minimizing the potential negative aspects of this treatment

(Ducruet, Zacharia et al. 2009). The addition of N-acetylheparin (a complement inhibitor) was found to significantly reduce cerebral edema at 24 and 72 h post-ICH in the same model. Subsequent studies have confirmed a central role for complement activation in the pathogenesis of ICH. Systemic depletion of complement using cobra venom factor (CVF) in rats resulted in significant reductions in perihematomal C9 deposition, C5a, TNF-α, myeloperoxidase (MPO)-positive cells, and C3d production, following ICH (Xi, Hua et al. 2001). Additionally, brain water measurements revealed a marked decrease in perihematomal edema (Xi, Hua et al. 2001). A study utilizing a similar nonspecific complement inhibitor, venom defibrase DF-521 batroxobin, confirmed these findings (Wu and Huang 2005). A potential role for the potent anaphylatoxin C5a in early edema formation and cerebral injury has also been suggested. Early studies once again utilized non-specific complement inhibitors and were therefore not able to precisely define the contribution of specific subcomponents of the complement cascade to injury after ICH. The recent advent of complement-deficient mice engendered a new phase of research in the pathogenesis of a wide variety of diseases. The first study employed C5-deficient mice in the setting of ICH and yielded surprising results. Relative to wild type C5-sufficent mice, C5-deficient animals demonstrated a significant increase in brain water content and greater neurologic impairment at 3 days following ICH (Nakamura, Xi et al. 2004).These paradoxic findings were explained by suggesting that activation of C5 may have a beneficial effect in this setting as demonstrated by Mukherjee and Pasinetti in a kainic acid-induced model of hippocampal damage, or perhaps that factors proximal to C5 are critical in mediating damage following ICH (Nakamura, Xi et al. 2004). Alternatively, C5-deficient mice might manifest unanticipated phenotypic compensation for the developmental lack of C5.

There is compelling animal data for an integral role for complement activation in mediating cerebral injury after ICH. Currently there are no effective pharmacological therapies for the treatment of ICH in humans. Selective and temporally targeted complement inhibition, particularly of C3, therefore represents an extremely attractive strategy for reducing inflammation, cerebral edema, and brain injury following human ICH, with the goal of improving functional outcomes (Ducruet, Zacharia et al. 2009).

2.2.3. Hemoglobin Intervention

Following intracerebral hemorrhage (ICH), the brain parenchyma is exposed to blood containing red blood cells (RBC) and consequently to its lysis products. Iron-rich hemoglobin (Hb) is the most abundant protein in RBC. The products of erythrocyte lyses, Hb and heme, are recognized as neurotoxins and the main contributors to delayed cerebral edema and tissue damage after intracerebral hemorrhage. Finding a means to efficiently control the detoxification and absorption of the hemolytic products (Hb and heme) is an important clinical challenge and critical for hematoma resolution. Clearance of cell-free Hb/heme through phagocytosis/endocytosis is an essential function of microglia/macrophages in anti-inflammatory response. When released into the brain parenchyma during hemolysis, Hb becomes a central mediator of cytotoxicity. Haptoglobin (Hp), an acute-phase response protein primarily synthesized in the liver and known to bind and neutralize Hb in the blood stream, is also expressed in brain where it plays an important role in defending neurons from damage induced by hemolytic products after ICH (Zhao, Song et al. 2009).

Haptoglobin (Hp) is a plasma protein and a key component of Hb detoxification system known for its role in conditions associated with intravascular hemolysis. Hp is an acute-phase α2-acid-response glycoprotein known to tightly bind Hb and form stable Hb-Hp complexes (Wada, Oara et al. 1970). Hp binds cell-free Hb to form essentially irreversible (Kd=1pM) Hp-Hb complexes, thereby blocking Hb-induced oxidative toxicity, enabling clearance of cell-free Hb and aiding in recycling of iron. By forming Hp-Hb complexes, Hp stabilizes and shields heme iron within the hydrophobic pocket of Hb, thereby preventing its pro-oxidative properties and cytotoxicity (Zuwala-Jagiello 2006). Hp is produced principally in liver by hepatocytes (Hoj, Binder et al. 1984) and secreted into blood circulation. The tissue-specific expression of Hp in some peripheral organs such as the lung, skin or kidney was demonstrated (Yang, Haile et al. 2003). Limited studies suggest the presence of Hp in neural retina, astrocytes after ischemia and subarachnoid blood clot, thus raising the speculation that under some conditions, in addition to its brain entry through disrupted blood-brain-barrier, Hp might be synthesized locally in the brain. As such, locally produced brain Hp may protect the brain from Hb-mediated damage in the case of ICH (Zhao, Song et al. 2009).

Hp reserves in blood plasma is normally relatively high to allows for efficient buffering of Hb in case of minor acute hemolytic events; however, serum levels of Hp can be dramatically increased in response to acute stress, inflammation and other pathological states, which improve efficiency of neutralization of free-Hb in case of severe hemolytic events. The timely binding of Hp to cell-free Hb plays an important role not only by blocking the pro-oxidative properties of Hb toward cellular constituents, but also toward Hb itself. The latter is particularly important since oxidatively modified Hb loses its binding affinity to Hp and CD163. Normally, when Hb is bound by Hp, the Hb-Hp complex supports structural stabilization of Hb and protects it from structural/oxidative modification. Otherwise, once the free Hb is oxidatively modified, Hp is no longer able to control its anti--oxidative properties and clearance through CD163-mediated endocytosis via macrophages (Buehler, Abraham et al. 2009).

Although the role of Hp in intravascular hemolysis is well-defined, its role in the brain and its expression by brain cells is essentially unknown. A recent study together with our present findings indicate that only very low Hp levels are present in the normal brain, thus contrasting with the high levels of Hp detected in the circulating blood and some peripheral organs. Interestingly, earlier experiments suggested that Hp expression could be induced in peripheral organs and not in the brain. For example, intraperitoneal injection of bacterial endotoxin was shown to cause robust increase in Hp expression in peripheral organs and blood serum, but not in the brain (D'Armiento, Dalal et al. 1997). This selective expression could be explained either by the distinct regulation of Hp expression in brain, or more likely by the fact that the signal triggering Hp expression in the periphery has no access to the normal brain. While induction of the peripheral Hp may occur without upregulation of the brain Hp, our present study indicates that selective brain damage by intracerebral injection of blood induces not only local (peri-hematoma) increase in brain's Hp mRNA and protein, but it also leads to a robust increase in Hp in peripheral blood. Interestingly, the expression profile of Hp in the brain follows the time-course of hemolysis-mediated cytotoxicity, peri-hematoma edema and tissue damage following ICH (Wagner and Dwyer 2004), suggesting that Hp may represent an endogenous factor normally involved in neutralization of hemolytic products toxicity in ICH-affected brain.

The role of oligodendroglia in Hp synthesis has not been suggested to date. Using in vivo and in vitro models of ICH, we have demonstrated here that brain's Hp is almost exclusively synthesized by oligodendrocytes. While some earlier studies suggested presence of Hp in the astroglia in hippocampus after global ischemia, blood clot in subarachnoid and in neutrophils, our present study failed to detect Hp in brain cells other than oligodendroglia after ICH. We consequently propose that oligodendrocytes which are known for their role in shielding and defending axons from excitotoxins and oxidative stress, could also protect axons from the damage imposed by hemolytic products via releasing Hb-neutralizing Hp into the periaxonal space. During intracerebral bleeding extravasated blood tends to spread along white matter tracts, where it may initiate direct toxicity to axons within the nerve tracts and therefore adversely affect neurological status. In agreement with this concept, mice overexpressing Hp showed better preservation of axonal integrity than Hp-null mice when subjected to ICH. Similarly, a reduced damage to neurofilament was observed in animals subjected to ICH and treated with sulforaphane (SF), the intervention associated with increased Hp expression, further supporting the evidence for an important role of Hp in protecting axons after ICH. Finally, oligodendroglia are also present in the gray matter where they could play protective role in context of lobar hemorrhage (Zhao, Song et al. 2009).

In summary, Hp is important for protecting brain from damage caused by ICH; Hp can be synthesized locally in the brain by oligodendroglia and released into the extracellular space where it can protect brain cells from damage mediated by hemolytic products. Hp plays a cytoprotective role after ICH, and Hp may represent a new potential therapeutic target for management of ICH (Zhao, Song et al. 2011).

2.2.4. Heme Intervention

Heme toxicity may contribute to the pathogenesis of intracerebral hemorrhage. The primary defense against extracellular heme is provided by hemopexin, a serum and neuronal glycoprotein that binds it with very high affinity and mitigates its prooxidant effect (Chen, Zhang et al. 2011). Hemopexin (Hx) is a blood plasma glycoprotein synthesized primarily by hepatocytes. Hx has been shown to bind to heme with a high affinity and forms stable Hx-heme complexs (Hvidberg, Maniecki et al. 2005, Wang, Manaenko et al. 2016). The heme-Hx complexes are readily endocytosed by macrophages expressing low-density lipoprotein receptor-related protein – LRP1 (α2-macroglobulin receptor, also known as CD91). While under physiological conditions LRP1 plays a role in recycling iron, in response to extravascular hemolysis in hematoma affected tissue, the Hx-heme/LRP1 system may facilitate removal of pro-oxidative heme by microglia/macrophages. Our study results demonstrated that recombinant LRP1 administration resulted in the raise of LPR1 positive cell number, which is a sign of the activation of heme–Hx clearance system. The activation of the heme–Hx system resulted in SOD1 upregulation and subsequently in the decrease of oxidative stress as well as attenuation of post-ICH apoptosis. This beneficial effects of LRP1 administration improved BBB integrity, resulted in the attenuation of brain edema formation and in the improvement of neurological functions (Wang, Manaenko et al. 2016). LRP1 may offer pleiotropic protective effects through promoting heme resolution and diminishing brain edema after ICH and may thus prove beneficial to post-ICH outcomes.

2.2.5. HO Modulation

The effects of an HO-1 inhibitor, tin-protoporphyrin (SnPP), attenuated hemoglobin-induced edema (Huang, Xi et al. 2002). Tin-mesoporphyrin (SnMP) is a neuroprotectant that has also been used clinically to treat hyperbilirubinemia. SnMP reduced intracerebral mass in an ICH model by decreasing both hematoma and edema volumes SnMP's mechanism of action is presently unknown but may involve its potent inhibition of heme oxygenase activity. Intravenous administration of nicaraven (a marked synergistic induction of HO-1 protein, for 2 days after subarachnoid hemorrhage) ameliorated delayed cerebral vasospasm in rat subarachnoid hemorrhage models. These results suggest that the enhanced HO-1 expression through a combination of pathological state and pharmacological agent could be an effective strategy to improve the prognosis of heme- and oxidative stress-induced diseases (Wang, Yang et al. 2011). Neuroprotective effects of Selective brain cooling (SBC) may be partially mediated by reducing the heme accumulation, which reduced injury-mediated upregulation of HO-1, and in turn ameliorated edema formation (Yao, Wei et al. 2011). Hemin treatment induced HO-1 protein expression and this was partially blocked by pretreatment with Valproic acid (VPA) (Kwon, Kim et al. 2013). Melatonin potentiates the neuroprotective effect of resveratrol (RSV) against oxidative injury, by enhancing HO-1 induction through inhibiting ubiquitination-dependent proteasome pathway (Kwon, Kim et al. 2011). So it's complicated to intervene HO and need consider the time window following ICH.

2.2.6. Iron Chelators

Iron derived from heme degradation may also play a key role in ICH pathogenesis, presumably via acceleration of oxidative stress. A recent clinical study showed that high serum levels of ferritin, a soluble protein for iron storage, are associated with poor outcome in ICH patients, suggesting that iron is involved in brain damage by ICH. Consistent with this results, several studies on animal models of ICH showed that the iron chelator deferoxamine attenuated tissue damage and neurological deficits. For instance, intraperitoneal administration of deferoxamine starting from 2 or 6 hours after autologous blood injection lessened brain edema, oxidative stress, and motor function deficits in rats. Another study on aged rats showed that deferoxamine was effective in reducing brain edema and motor dysfunctioneven when administration of the drug was delayed 12and 48 h, respectively, after autologous blood injection. However, the therapeutic efficacy of deferoxamine might depend on the type of ICH model. Reports mentioned above demonstrating beneficial effects of deferoxamine are based on the model made by autologous blood injection, whereas deferoxamine did not improve the outcome of the collagenase-induced ICH model in rats. On the other hand, a study on clioquinol, another kind of metal chelator, has demonstrated that oral administration of the drug, starting 6 h after induction of hemorrhage near the internal capsule by collagenase, alleviatedmotor dysfunction of rats (Katsuki 2010). Ferric iron chelators such as deferoxamine and deferiprone lowered iron deposition in brain following ICH (Wang, Hu et al. 2015, He, Lan et al. 2016), However ferric iron chelation does not improve the outcome after ICH (Auriat, Silasi et al. 2012). Clioquinol, a ferrous iron chelator, improved the neurological outcome, attenuated brain edema, and ROS production besides reducing iron levels in our study(Wang, Hu et al. 2015). Another ferrous chelator, 2,2'-bipyridine, is a potential means of ameliorating iron-induced injury after ICH (Wu, Wu et al. 2012), unfortunately another results failed to support the use of bipyridine against ICH (Caliaperumal, Wowk et al. 2013), the function of bipyridine on ICH is uncertain so far.

Our study results demonstrated that ferrous iron may play a key role in the pathogenesis of secondary injury after ICH. Fe^{2+} binding may attenuate some ROS consequences from iron overload then mitigate brain edema. Exogenous iron chelator functioned by affecting endogenous iron chelators or transporters. Clioquinol improved neurological outcome of rat ICH probably through reducing brain edema and ROS production, it facilitated Fe^{2+} export and inhibited Fe^{2+} import through enhancing Fpn and reducing divalentmetal transport 1 (DMT1) expression. Deferiprone failed to improve the outcome probably owing to its upregulation for DMT1 but nothing to ferroportin, so deferiprone seemed to have little effect on brain edema and ROS (Wang, Hu et al. 2015).

2.2.7. Bilirubin Inhibitor

Toxicity and damage from bilirubin in vitro and in vivo was prevented by dimethyl sulfoxide (Lakovic, Ai et al. 2014). So Dimethyl sulfoxide or its derivatives may have a potential therapeutic role at antagonizing axonal damage after hemorrhagic stroke (Lakovic, Ai et al. 2014). Minocycline, an anti-inflammatory and anti-apoptotic semisynthetic tetracycline, can prevent hyperbilirubinemia-induced cerebellar hypoplasia in Gunn rats (Geiger, Rice et al. 2007). Sn-mesoporphyrin (SnMP), a potent inhibitor of bilirubin production, can mitigate neonatal hyperbilirubinemia (Valaes, Drummond et al. 1998) and be neuroprotective that has also been used clinically to treat hyperbilirubinemia (Wagner, Hua et al. 2000).

2.2.8. Antioxidants and Free Radical Scavengers

Experimental studies have confirmed that oxidative stress plays a pivotal role in cerebral injury following ICH. The amount of oxidative DNA is increased after ICH in the animal model, and administration of a free radical scavenger, edaravone suppressed DNA oxidation and brain damage after ICH (Hama, Ishihara et al. 2012). The oxidative products of macromolecules significantly increased, whereas antioxidant enzymes, such as superoxide dismutase (SOD), glutathione peroxidase (GPx), and catalase, correspondingly decreased as a result of ICH (Nakamura, Keep et al. 2005, Nakamura, Keep et al. 2006). Free radical scavengers proved to be effective in neuroprotection in animal ICH models.

Repeated treatment with the lower dose of melatonin (5 mg/kg) given at 1 h and every 24 h thereafter for 3 days after ICH, led to normalization of striatal function and memory ability over the course of 8 weeks, and less brain atrophy 2 weeks later. These results suggest that melatonin is safe for use after ICH, reduces oxidative stress, provides brain protection, and could be used for future investigations of free radical mechanisms after cerebral hemorrhage (Lekic, Hartman et al. 2010).

Sulfaphenazole (SPZ) has a different mechanism such as reactive oxygen species scavenging, in addition to the inhibition of superoxide production by cytochrome P450. The results showed that systemic SPZ treatment after intracerebral hemorrhage reduces striatal dysfunction, the elevation of lipid peroxidation, and brain edema in the rat. These results suggest that SPZ is a potentially effective therapeutic approach for intracerebral hemorrhage as the effect of SPZ was initiated for either 1 h or 3 d post-intracerebral hemorrhage (Hama, Ishihara et al. 2012). SPZ inhibited lipid peroxidation in the ipsilateral region, thus suggesting that brain damage could be suppressed by the reduction of oxidative stress by SPZ, but not due to CYP inhibition by SPZ. Superoxide anion is converted to hydrogen peroxide via dismutation catalyzed by superoxide dismutase, followed by production of hydroxyl radicals in the presence of iron ion. Hydroxyl radical production could be facilitated in the localization of bleeding because there is excess iron in a hematoma or its distal region. SPZ might therefore suppress the chain-reaction of ROS causing tissue oxidation and injury via brain edema. Therefore, SPZ is considered to have a beneficial effect on the behavioral outcomes following ICH, thus suggesting that ROS scavenging, but not the CYP2C family, plays at least some type of role in the development of brain damage following ICH. In addition, the next step is to investigate the mechanism (s) of action of SPZ on brain damage after ICH (Hama, Ishihara et al. 2012). However, no antioxidant has been applied in patients with ICH because of the unclear mechanism of OS-related injury. The current review attempted to illustrate the knowledge regarding ICH-related OS and its possible molecular mechanism and to discuss the potential targets of intervention for future research.

Angiotensin II is a potent vasoconstrictor hormone that is cleaved from angiotensinogen by renin and angiotensin-converting enzyme, which also is the principal inducer of oxidative stress and inflammation. The acute blockade of AT1R might exert beneficial effects in the hemorrhagic brain. ARBs were also proven to attenuate inflammatory and oxidative stress and to regulate the nitric-oxide synthase isoenzymes in the brain. As a potent and highly selective AT1 receptor antagonist, telmisartan (TMS) is described chemically as 4[(1,4-dimethyl-2-propyl[2,6-bi-1H-benzimidazol]-1-yl)methyl] [1,1-biphenyl]-2-carboxylic acid. This unique feature of telmisartan accounts for both its high receptor affinity and its excellent pharmacokinetic properties. Furthermore, telmisartan could confer effects other than the blockage of the AT1R, such as peroxisome proliferator-activated receptor (PPAR) γ activation. Telmisartan reduced hemorrhage volume, brain edema, and inflammatory or apoptotic cells in the perihematomal area. Telmisartan was noted to induce the expression of endothelial nitric-oxide synthase and peroxisome proliferator-activated receptor γ and decrease oxidative stress, apoptotic signal, tumor necrosis factor-α, and cyclooxygenase-2 expression. The telmisartan-treated rats exhibited less pronounced neurological deficits and recovered better. Thus, telmisartan seems to offer neural protection, including antiapoptosis, anti-inflammatory, and antioxidant benefits in the intracerebral hemorrhage rat model (Jung, Chu et al. 2007).

The administration of the antioxidant compound U-74389G, results in early decrease of inflammatory response following ICH (Bimpis, Papalois et al. 2015). Edaravone, a novel synthetic small-molecule free-radical scavenger, has been shown a neuroprotection in both animal models of cerebral ischemia and stroke patients (Wang, Jiang et al. 2011) bypreventing oxidative stress and blood brain barrier damage (Lukic-Panin, Deguchi et al. 2010). Alpha-Lipoic acid improved longer-term memory of aged mice based on its free radical scavenger properties (Stoll, Hartmann et al. 1993). Carvedilol, a new vasodilator and beta adrenoceptor antagonist, inhibits lipid peroxidation mainly via scavenging free radicals (Yue, Cheng et al. 1992).

CONCLUSION

The secondary insults after primary intracerebral hemorrhage is believed to be mediated by the cytotoxic, excitotoxic, oxidative, and inflammatory effects of intraparenchymal blood. The main factors responsible for this injury are thrombin and erythrocyte components such as hemoglobin, heme, iron and bilirubin. Therapies including thrombin inhibitors, antiinflammatory drugs, antagonists for hemoglobin, heme and bilirubin, chelators to bind free iron are currently under investigation for reducing this secondary brain injury. This chapter discussed the molecular mechanisms of brain injury as a result of intraparenchymal blood, potential targets for therapeutic intervention, and treatment strategies currently in development.

Chapter 2

HEMATOMA EXPANSION: CLINICAL AND MOLECULAR PREDICTORS AND CORRESPONDING PHARMACOLOGICAL TREATMENT

ABSTRACT

The secondary insultsafterintracerebral hemorrhage (ICH) mainly occurs as a result of hematoma expansion. So prevention from hematoma expansion is essential to reduce deleterious pathological process and improve clinical outcomes in patients suffering from ICH. In this chapter, available information of hematoma expansion from clinical signs to molecular mechanisms are provided and potential intervention strategies discussed. We introduced all possible risk biomarkers of hematoma expansion, such as coagulation/hemostasis dysfunction, higher blood pressure and BRAIN scores, higher serum glucose and/or glycosylated hemoglobin A1c, serum creatinine, Factor XIII and international normalized ratio (INR), lower serum cholesterol or LDL cholesterol, and fibrinogen. Furthermore, there are several molecular pathways (i.e., plasma kallikrein, von Willebrand factor, N-methyl-D-aspartate and its receptor, cytokines/ adipokines, cellular fibronectin and apolipoprotein Eε2 allele) may lead to hematoma expansion. We discussed the forementioned predictors and provided corresponding treatments to prevent occurance of hematoma expansion (Wang and Zhang 2016).

INTRODUCTION

Intracerebral hemorrhage (ICH), the most devastating form of stroke, has no specific therapy proven to improve outcome by randomized controlled trial. Location and baseline hematoma volume are strong predictors of mortality, but are non-modifiable by the time of diagnosis. Expansion of the initial hematoma is a further marker of poor prognosis that may be at least partly preventable. Hematoma expansion is so far the only marker of outcome that is amenable to treatment and thus a potentially important therapeutic target (Brouwers and Greenberg 2013).

Hematoma volume at presentation, further increase of hematoma volume, and the development of intraventricular hemorrhage were shown to be independent predictors of poor outcome, and hematoma growth (as defined by Brott et al. see subsequently) was also found to be a predictor of early neurological deterioration. These findings indicate that early extension of the initial hematoma boundaries has substantial clinical implications. Increase of hematoma volume is a frequent complication in ICH and was observed in >70% of cases when defined as any increase in parenchymal volume or intraventricular invasion (Steiner and Bosel 2010).Hematoma expansion is the primary cause of neurologic deterioration after intracerebral hemorrhage (Kazui, Minematsu et al. 1997, Xi, Keep et al. 2006, Sahni and Weinberger 2007) and remains one of the few remediable risk factors for poor outcome (Tsai, Hsu et al. 2011, Appelboom, Piazza et al. 2013). Early restriction of intracerebral hemorrhage is of paramount importance because secondary volume expansion leads to outcome deterioration and death. Hematoma expansion occurs in about one third of patients with cerebral hemorrhage (Kazui, Minematsu et al. 1997, Xi, Keep et al. 2006, Pandey and Xi 2014). In a study by Brott and colleagues, hematoma growth was defined by an increase in hematoma volume by 33% of the baseline volume (Morotti, Jessel et al. 2016), i.e., a 10% increase in diameter (Brott, Broderick et al. 1997, Cheung 1998, Li, Huang et al. 2015).

An almost linear association between hematoma expansion and the probability of poor outcome has been reported: a 1 mL additional hematoma expansion yields a 5% increased risk of death and dependency (Delcourt, Huang et al. 2012, Ovesen, Havsteen et al. 2014). Hematoma expansion is a significant, independent predictor of adverse outcomes after ICH, over and above established baseline prognostic indicators (Davis, Broderick et al. 2006, Ovesen, Havsteen et al. 2014). Therefore, effective therapy directed at stopping rebleeding in acute ICH patients could potentially decrease mortality and improve the neurological outcome (Pandey and Xi 2014). Therefore, additional information on the precise underlying mechanisms of hematoma expansion and its potential therapeutic interventions is required.

The pathophysiology behind early hematoma expansion is not well understood. It is not clear whether it reflects leakage, rebleeding, or both. Several mechanisms of brain injury after SICH have been investigated, but most of these evolve too late to account for early hematoma expansion. In addition to disruption of supportive and protective functional tissue, elevated intracranial pressure, reduced oxygen supply, and mitochondrial dysfunction in the perihematomal zone, deleterious factors in the blood or perihematomal edema might act on vessels and the blood–brain barrier. Animal and human studies suggest an association of inflammatory activation (increased interleukin-6, tumor necrosis factor-α) and degradation of components of the blood–brain barrier basal membrane (e.g., fibronectins) by matrix metalloproteinases with hematoma enlargement in SICH. Furthermore, repeated or continuous bleeding can be the result of coagulopathies or anticoagulants. A role for disturbed autoregulation and uncontrolled perfusion pressure in hypertension as a driving force of further bleeding is conceivable, but data on this are controversial (Steiner and Bosel 2010).

This part focuses on the current understanding of the mechanisms underlying hematoma expansion and proposes potential strategies for clinical prevention and intervention.

1. Terminology and Definition of Hematoma Expansion

Terms for the phenomenon of hematoma enlargement in SICH have not been used consistently in the literature. They include growth, enlargement, extension, expansion, rebleeding, and so on. Here we adopted the definition [2] of hematoma expansion as all forms of extended spatial distribution of the initial hemorrhage, including intraparenchymal volume enlargement, invasion of the ventricles (not necessarily associated with change in intraparenchymal volume), transition or rebleeding into compartments (such as the subarachnoid space) adjacent to the side of the original hemorrhage. It didn't include the formation of perihematomal edema in this definition, although this may play a role in the pathophysiology of hematoma expansion. Early hematoma expansion as hematoma expansion occurring within the first 24 hours after onset of SICH, that is, the vast majority of all relevant hematoma expansions. The efforts to restrict hematoma expansion as all measures that are undertaken to prevent or reduce hematoma expansion in the first place. This does not include treating the consequences of hematoma expansion such as lowering intracranial pressure, hematoma evacuation merely aimed at volume reduction, or clearance of the ventricles.

These definitions are used throughout this chapter. This part is focused on prevention or attenuation of early hematoma expansion, not on the sequelae and complications beyond 24 hours, which will be discussed in Part 2. Here, we summarize the risk factors of hematoma expansion, present current knowledge on surgical and nonsurgical approaches toward hematoma expansion, and finally outline future strategies (Steiner and Bosel 2010).

2. Predictors of Hematoma Expansion

Many predictors of hematoma expansion (Figure 3) have been proposed, but some of them e.g., fibrinogen (Fujii, Takeuchi et al. 1998, Marti-Fabregas, Borrell et al. 2010), blood pressure (Fujii, Takeuchi et al. 1998, Davis, Broderick et al. 2006, Jauch, Lindsell et al. 2006, Pandey and Xi 2014, Gioia, Kate et al. 2015, Wang, Arima et al. 2015), blood glucose (Kazui, Minematsu et al. 1997, Davis, Broderick et al. 2006, Broderick, Diringer et al. 2007, Liu, Gao et al. 2011), and IVH (Cheung 1998, Silva, Leira et al. 2005, Albright, Burak et al. 2013, Wang, Arima et al. 2015) remain controversial.

In patients with medical histories of bleeding and/or coagulation abnormalities (Schlunk, Schulz et al. 2015), who suffered from liver disease (Kazui, Minematsu et al. 1997) and/or were alcoholics (Fujii, Takeuchi et al. 1998), who were under treatment of anticoagulants (Huttner, Schellinger et al. 2006, Emiru, Bershad et al. 2013, Hanger, Geddes et al. 2013, James, Palys et al. 2013, Le Roux, Pollack et al. 2014, Yaghi, Eisenberger et al. 2014, Schlunk, Schulz et al. 2015) or antiplatelets (Broderick, Diringer et al. 2007, Naidech, Jovanovic et al. 2009, James, Palys et al. 2013) (i.e, for valvular heart disease, venous thromboembolism and/or atrial fibrillation (Stampfli, Asmis et al. 2008, Kuramatsu, Gerner et al. 2015, Ruff, Giugliano et al. 2015) , and brain infarction (Kazui, Minematsu et al. 1997)) or where there was prior ICH, the odds of hematoma expansion were higher. A coagulation/ hemostasis dysfunction appears to contribute to hematoma growth.

Other clinical predictors include higher blood pressure (BP) on admission (systolic BP $\geqslant$ 160-200mmHg) (Kazui, Minematsu et al. 1997, Fujii,

Takeuchi et al. 1998, Ohwaki, Yano et al. 2004, Lim, Hwang et al. 2008, Rodriguez-Luna, Pineiro et al. 2013, Takeda, Ogura et al. 2013, Kuramatsu, Gerner et al. 2015), higher BRAIN scores (Wang, Arima et al. 2015)based on Baseline ICH volume, Recurrent ICH, Anticoagulation with warfarin at onset, Intraventricular extension, and the Number of hours to baseline CT from symptom onset (Chan and Hemphill 2014, Morawo and Gilmore 2016). The larger volume of ICH (Ohwaki, Yano et al. 2004, Broderick, Diringer et al. 2007, Takeda, Ogura et al. 2013, Kuramatsu, Gerner et al. 2015), the shorter time period from symptom onset to CT (Fujii, Takeuchi et al. 1998, Wang, Arima et al. 2015) , as well as Recurrent ICH, Anticoagulation with warfarin at onset, Intraventricular extension (Brott, Broderick et al. 1997, Huttner, Schellinger et al. 2006, Xi, Keep et al. 2006, Yaghi, Dibu et al. 2014, Wang, Arima et al. 2015, Morawo and Gilmore 2016), predicted a higher risk of hematoma expansion (Wang, Arima et al. 2015). The BRAIN scores can be easily assessed and implemented by clinicians and, in particular, can be used for shared clinical decision-making where CTA is not readily available or routinely performed for acute ICH (Wang, Arima et al. 2015). In addition, it was reported that consciousness disturbance on admission (Fujii, Takeuchi et al. 1998) and less mass index (Broderick, Diringer et al. 2007) were more likely to cause hematoma growth.

Where laboratory indices included higher serum glucose (Kazui, Minematsu et al. 1997, Broderick, Diringer et al. 2007, Liu, Gao et al. 2011, Qureshi, Palesch et al. 2011)and/or glycosylated hemoglobin A1c (Kazui, Minematsu et al. 1997), higher serum creatinine (Broderick, Diringer et al. 2007), Factor XIII (Marti-Fabregas, Borrell et al. 2010) and international normalized ratio (INR) (Le Roux, Pollack et al. 2014, Pandey and Xi 2014, Kuramatsu, Gerner et al. 2015), lower serum cholesterol (Broderick, Diringer et al. 2007) or LDL cholesterol (Rodriguez-Luna, Rubiera et al. 2011), and fibrinogen (Fujii, Takeuchi et al. 1998), the chances of expanding hematomas were greater.

Patients with imaging characteristics displaying irregularly shaped hematoma (Fujii, Takeuchi et al. 1998), hematoma heterogeneity (Takeda, Ogura et al. 2013) , spot sign on computed tomography angiography (CTA) (Goldstein, Fazen et al. 2007, Wada, Aviv et al. 2007, Delgado Almandoz, Yoo et al. 2010, Demchuk, Dowlatshahi et al. 2012, Ovesen, Havsteen et al. 2014, Radmanesh, Falcone et al. 2014), and intraventricular hemorrhage (IVH) and/or extension (Cheung 1998, Wang, Arima et al. 2015) were at an increased risk of hematoma expansion. The so-called "spot-sign," which reflects contrast extravasation into the hematoma, has increasingly gained attention, and many studies have included this parameter to promote recognition of a potential target population in hematoma expansion prevention (Goldstein, Fazen et al. 2007, Wada, Aviv et al. 2007, Radmanesh, Falcone et al. 2014, Morotti, Jessel et al. 2016, Wang and Zhang 2016).

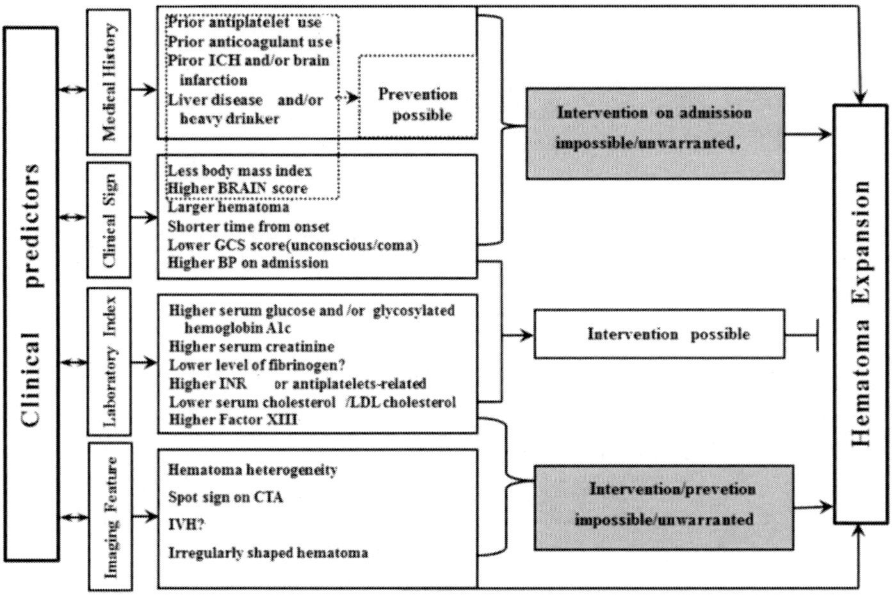

Figure 3. Clinical markers (medical history, clinical signs on admission, laboratory and imaging findings) could predict to hematoma expansion and potential intervention.

3. Current Clinical Prevention of Hematoma Expansion

Risk of hematoma expansion may be alleviated by premorbid management of liver disease, alcohol consumption, and prior infarct (Kazui, Minematsu et al. 1997). Controlling daily alcohol consumption or abstaining from alcohol may serve to lower the risk of hematoma growth. It is known that controlling blood pressure (BP) is beneficial for preventing recurrent stroke (hemorrhagic and ischemic) (Rashid, Leonardi-Bee et al. 2003, Fuentes, Ortega-Casarrubios et al. 2007, De Lima, Saconato et al. 2014, Pandey and Xi 2014, Steiner, Al-Shahi Salman et al. 2014, Sherzai and Elkind 2015).

However, because there are many other etiologies that cause ICH and ischemic stroke, only controlling BP is not enough to prevent stroke recurrence.

Current guidelines recommend antiplatelet therapy for non-cardioembolic ischemic stroke or TIA, with aspirin, clopidogrel, or their combination for prevention of stroke recurrence (Albers and Amarenco 2001, Shulga and Bornstein 2011, Aw and Sharma 2012, Kernan, Ovbiagele et al. 2014, Sherzai and Elkind 2015). Clopidogrel may be used as an alternative to aspirin–dypiridamole for secondary stroke prevention (Shulga and Bornstein 2011, Aw and Sharma 2012, Kernan, Ovbiagele et al. 2014, Sherzai and Elkind 2015). For decades warfarin has been used to lower the risk of stroke in patients with atrial fibrillation. Previous studies indicated that dose-adjusted warfarin significantly reduced the incidence of stroke, but its use is associated with risk of bleeding (Hsu, Hsieh et al. 2015) and/or rebleeding (Turpie 2008, Cairns, Connolly et al. 2011, Pandey and Xi 2014, Hsu, Hsieh et al. 2015). Paradoxically, warfarin may be a way to prevent brain ischemic stroke and cause lower hematoma expansion, because hematoma expansion is common in the setting of anticoagulant-related (Huttner, Schellinger et al. 2006, Emiru, Bershad et al. 2013, Hanger, Geddes et al. 2013, James, Palys et al. 2013, Le Roux, Pollack et al. 2014, Yaghi, Eisenberger et al. 2014, Schlunk, Schulz et al. 2015) and antiplatelets-related (Broderick, Diringer et al. 2007, Naidech, Jovanovic et al. 2009, James, Palys et al. 2013) ICH. It is necessary that patients on warfarin or antiplatelets therapy be periodically monitored with dose adjustments.

Another preventable index is body mass index (BMI), with patients having higher BMIs at a lesser risk of hematoma expansion (Broderick, Diringer et al. 2007). The author explained that this may be due to a volume-based dose relationship of rFVIIa, which was administered based on estimated body weight (Ribo and Grotta 2006, Broderick, Diringer et al. 2007). It may also be related to the reduced lipid level (Broderick, Diringer et al. 2007, Rodriguez-Luna, Rubiera et al. 2011) from the lower BMI. This phenomenon may demonstrate that an improved nutritional status and energy reservoirs serve as protections against mortality, and that following a healthy lifestyle may reduce adverse outcomes associated with obesity in patients with higher BMIs (Bagheri, Speakman et al. 2015).

4. Therapeutic Options to Restrict Hematoma Expansion

To date, no individual treatment for ICH has shown benefit in a randomized controlled trial, although specialized treatment provided by a neuroscience ICU does appear to reduce mortality (Diringer and Edwards 2001, Brouwers and Greenberg 2013). Because of its strong relationship with outcome and the potential to alter its course, hematoma expansion is an appealing therapeutic target. Therapeutic options to restrict hematoma expansion can be divided into surgical and nonsurgical approaches, whereas the 2 might complement each other.

4.1. Surgical Approach

With respect to the restriction of hematoma expansion, neurosurgical intervention can have the following aims: removal of the source of hemorrhage, staunching of the bleeding, and elimination of the effects of blood degradation products. The mere removal of blood by open craniotomy or stereotactic aspiration, that is, reduction of mass, cannot be regarded as a measure to restrict hematoma expansion. Although it could be argued that the removal of blood leads to elimination of deleterious promotors of further bleeding or allows access to a bleeding source, these aspects were not looked at or reported specifically in most of the relevant surgical trials performed so far. Another problem is that most surgical trials did not identify early hematoma expansion or enroll enough patients early enough to allow conclusions on restriction in the sense of our definitions. Morgenstern and coworkers performed 2 small trials to answer the question of intervention timing. Indeed, the first study revealed better outcome for those patients operated within 12 hours after onset (Morgenstern, Frankowski et al. 1998). However, the follow-up study with a time window of 4 hours showed a higher mortality due to an increased rebleeding rate (Morgenstern, Demchuk et al. 2001). However, it is not clear whether early hematoma expansion had an influence on these results. Release of tamponating tissue pressure at this early stage of the disease may have caused rebleeding. Some authors therefore consider a combination of hemostatics with early surgery a promising alternative (2005). The Surgical Trial in IntraCerebral Hemorrhage (STICH), currently the largest prospective trial on surgery in SICH, that failed to show an outcome benefit over conservative treatment, cannot be applied to the question of early hematoma expansion restriction either; with a time window of 96 hours, mean time from ictus to surgery was 30 hours, that is, after the majority of relevant hematoma expansions should already have occurred. Furthermore, hematoma expansion was not specifically identified and surgical treatment (craniotomy in 75%) was mainly directed at reduction of mass and pressure. STICH-II, the follow-up trial limited to patients with lobar ICH without intraventricular hemorrhage, will probably not answer the question of surgical hematoma expansion restriction either because of a similar time window (Mendelow and Unterberg 2007). More interesting with regard to hematoma expansion might be endoscopic surgery, because iatrogenic bleeding risk might be reduced in an early, less stable phase of ICH and the coagulation of oozing vessels can be combined with hematoma evacuation. Evidence, however, is very limited; 20 years ago, a small prospective randomized trial of endoscopic versus medical treatment of 100 patients with SICH resulted in better outcome and reduced mortality for endoscopic treatment within 48 hour of onset (Auer, Deinsberger et al. 1989). More recently, Cho and colleagues introduced a score for basal ganglia hemorrhage and evaluated its prediction power in endoscopic versus conservative treatment of 226 patients (Cho, Chen et al. 2008). The authors concluded that a midlevel modified intracerebral hemorrhage score of 2 to 4 (based on the determinants Glasgow Coma Score, intracerebral hemorrhage volume, and intraventricular hemorrhage or hydrocephalus) favors endoscopic surgery to improve function or reduce mortality. Unfortunately, due to differences in surgical technique, radiological documentation, and timing of treatment in the aforementioned surgical trials, it is difficult, if not impossible, to draw any conclusions on hematoma expansion restriction. In fact, evidence that surgery alone can restrict expansion of ICH is presently not existent. Clearly, trials that are tailored more individually with regard to patient characteristics and ICH features are still necessary to elucidate the role of surgery (Steiner and Bosel 2010). To date, surgery might add to medical treatment with regard to survival or independence, but this is not very robust, and thus, no general recommendation can be given with regard to surgical prevention of hematoma expansion (Prasad, Mendelow et al. 2008, Steiner and Bosel 2010).

Surgical interventions have not been proven beneficial in randomized controlled trials, with the exception of cerebellar ICH (van Loon, Van Calenbergh et al. 1993). Minimally invasive surgical techniques also provide promising evidence for future surgical treatment options in acute ICH (Newell, Shah et al. 2011). It remains unclear whether the possible benefits of surgical clot removal are related to preventing subsequent expansion, or rather to reduced pathogenic effects of the clot itself such as mass effect or neurotoxicity related to hemoglobin, thrombin, and iron accumulation (Brouwers and Greenberg 2013).

4.2. Potential Clinical Nonsurgical Intervention for Hematoma Expansion

Several medical therapies have been studied in randomized controlled trials over the last decades. Some of the clinical signs and nearly all of the laboratory findings indicate that hematoma expansion can be intervened (Figure 3 and Figure 4) (Wang and Zhang 2016).

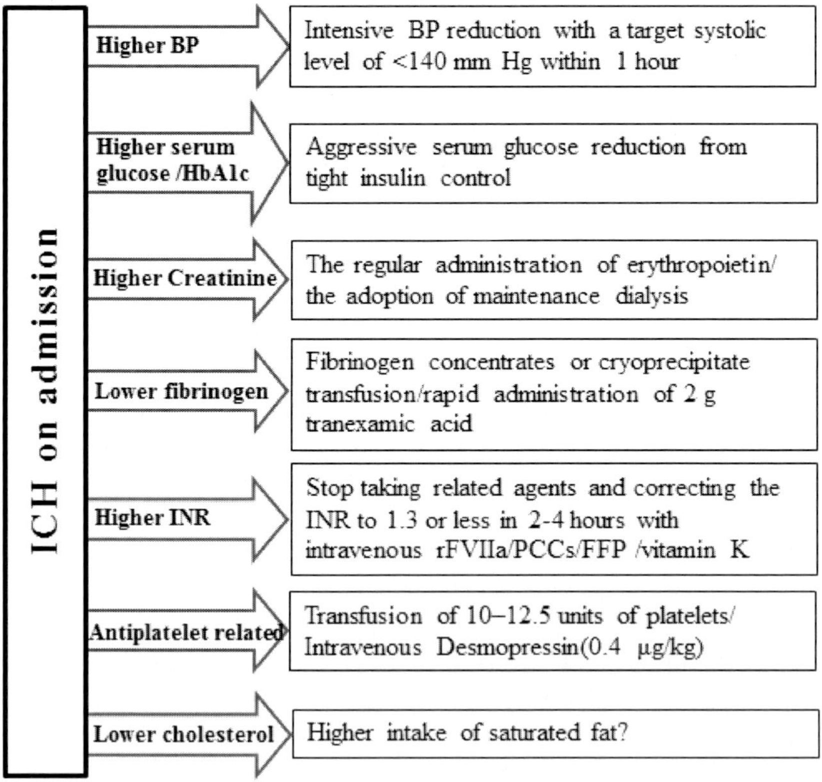

Figure 4. Avaliable clinical intervention measures to block hematoma expansion in detail.

4.2.1. Blood Pressure Modulation

Higher blood pressures (Kazui, Minematsu et al. 1997, Fujii, Takeuchi et al. 1998, Ohwaki, Yano et al. 2004, Anderson, Huang et al. 2008, Lim, Hwang et al. 2008, Takeda, Ogura et al. 2013, Pandey and Xi 2014, Kuramatsu, Gerner et al. 2015) have been recognized to increase hematoma expansion (Kazui, Minematsu et al. 1997, Fujii, Takeuchi et al. 1998, Ohwaki, Yano et al. 2004, Anderson, Huang et al. 2008, Lim, Hwang et al. 2008, Takeda, Ogura et al. 2013, Pandey and Xi 2014, Kuramatsu, Gerner et al. 2015), although precise data on the risks and benefits of acute BP lowering remain limited (Davis, Broderick et al. 2006, Jauch, Lindsell et al. 2006, Kuramatsu, Huttner et al. 2013, Gioia, Kate et al. 2015, Wang, Arima et al. 2015). The INTERACT I and ATACH I pilot studies revealed a safety profile and lower risk of hematoma expansion when aggressive systolic BP lowering to levels between 110–140 mmHg was achieved (Anderson, Huang et al. 2008, Kawanishi, Kawai et al. 2008, Kuramatsu, Huttner et al. 2013). More specifically, the Intensive Blood Pressure Reduction in INTERACT II has evaluated the safety and efficacy of intensive BP reduction (Tsivgoulis and Katsanos 2015) (with a target systolic level of <140 mmHg within 1 hour) in comparison to guideline-recommended BP treatment (with a target systolic level of <180 mm Hg) (Anderson, Heeley et al. 2013)and has shown a favorable trend toward improved functional outcomes with intensive BP reduction (Anderson, Heeley et al. 2013, Pandey and Xi 2014). Together with INTERACT, the results form the basis for a larger randomized trial to compare intensive (target SBP <140 mmHg) with standard (target SBP <180 mmHg) treatment by intravenous nicardipine within 3 hours. Feasibility of intensive blood pressure reduction below a mean arterial pressure of 110 mmHg was also reported in a smaller prospective controlled trial of 42 patients with ICH (Koch, Romano et al. 2008). Moreover, intensive BP reduction appears to be associated with a greater attenuation of absolute hematoma growth at 24 hours (Tsivgoulis, Katsanos et al. 2014).

Appreciating a slight effect of antihypertensives on hematoma expansion reduction in an overall weak or equivocal context of evidence and considering that (1) autoregulation is often preserved in the acute phase (as opposed to the postacute phase) of ICH; and (2) aggressive lowering of blood pressure theoretically carries the risk of cerebral ischemia in hypertensive patients, it seems reasonable to presently follow current guidelines and lower blood pressure cautiously (Broderick, Connolly et al. 2007).

Although INTERACT2 demonstrated consistency of the treatment effect across several prespecified patient subgroups, there was no clear relationship between outcome and the time from onset of ICH to commencing treatment and no significant effect of intensive BP-lowering treatment on hematoma growth. Moreover, only one third of patients achieved the target SBP level within 1 hour (half achieved the target by 6 hours), and most (75%) presented with mild to moderate size (<20 mmHg) on presentation, large and more severe ICH, and those requiring surgical decompression. Because the speed and degree of BP reduction will vary according to the agent and method of delivery (bolus versus infusion) and clinical features, the choice of agent should take into account the practicability, pharmacological profile, potential side effects, and cost (Hemphill, Greenberg et al. 2015).

Table 1. Applying Classification of Recommendations and Level of Evidence

SIZE OF TREATMENT EFFECT

ESTIMATE OF CERTAINTY (PRECISION) OF TREATMENT EFFECT	CLASS I *Benefit >>> Risk* Procedure/Treatment **SHOULD** be performed/ administered	CLASS IIa *Benefit >> Risk* *Additional studies with focused objectives needed* **IT IS REASONABLE** to perform procedure/administer treatment	CLASS IIb *Benefit ≥ Risk* *Additional studies with broad objectives needed; additional registry data would be helpful* Procedure/Treatment **MAY BE CONSIDERED**	CLASS III *No Benefit* or CLASS III *Harm* COR III: No benefit — Procedure/Test: Not Helpful; Treatment: No Proven Benefit COR III: Harm — Procedure/Test: Excess Cost w/o Benefit or Harmful; Treatment: Harmful to Patients
LEVEL A Multiple populations evaluated* Data derived from multiple randomized clinical trials or meta-analyses	■ Recommendation that procedure or treatment is useful/effective ■ Sufficient evidence from multiple randomized trials or meta-analyses	■ Recommendation in favor of treatment or procedure being useful/effective ■ Some conflicting evidence from multiple randomized trials or meta-analyses	■ Recommendation's usefulness/efficacy less well established ■ Greater conflicting evidence from multiple randomized trials or meta-analyses	■ Recommendation that procedure or treatment is not useful/effective and may be harmful ■ Sufficient evidence from multiple randomized trials or meta-analyses
LEVEL B Limited populations evaluated* Data derived from a single randomized trial or nonrandomized studies	■ Recommendation that procedure or treatment is useful/effective ■ Evidence from single randomized trial or nonrandomized studies	■ Recommendation in favor of treatment or procedure being useful/effective ■ Some conflicting evidence from single randomized trial or nonrandomized studies	■ Recommendation's usefulness/efficacy less well established ■ Greater conflicting evidence from single randomized trial or nonrandomized studies	■ Recommendation that procedure or treatment is not useful/effective and may be harmful ■ Evidence from single randomized trial or nonrandomized studies
LEVEL C Very limited populations evaluated* Only consensus opinion of experts, case studies, or standard of care	■ Recommendation that procedure or treatment is useful/effective ■ Only expert opinion, case studies, or standard of care	■ Recommendation in favor of treatment or procedure being useful/effective ■ Only diverging expert opinion, case studies, or standard of care	■ Recommendation's usefulness/efficacy less well established ■ Only diverging expert opinion, case studies, or standard of care	■ Recommendation that procedure or treatment is not useful/effective and may be harmful ■ Only expert opinion, case studies, or standard of care
Suggested phrases for writing recommendations	should is recommended is indicated is useful/effective/beneficial	is reasonable can be useful/effective/beneficial is probably recommended or indicated	may/might be considered may/might be reasonable usefulness/effectiveness is unknown/unclear/uncertain or not well established	COR III: No Benefit: is not recommended; is not indicated; should not be performed/ administered/ other; is not useful/ beneficial/ effective COR III: Harm: potentially harmful; causes harm; associated with excess morbidity/mortality; should not be performed/ administered/ other
Comparative effectiveness phrases†	treatment/strategy A is recommended/indicated in preference to treatment B treatment A should be chosen over treatment B	treatment/strategy A is probably recommended/indicated in preference to treatment B it is reasonable to choose treatment A over treatment B		

Table 2. Definition of Classes and Levels of Evidence Used inAHA/ASA Recommendations

Definition of Classes and Levels of Evidence Used in AHA Stroke Council Recommendations

Class I	Conditions for which there is evidence for and/or general agreement that the procedure or treatment is useful and effective.	
Class II	Conditions for which there is conflicting evidence and/or a divergence of opinion about the usefulness/efficacy of a procedure or treatment.	
	Class IIa	The weight of evidence or opinion is in favor of the procedure or treatment.
	Class IIb	Usefulness/efficacy is less well established by evidence or opinion.
Class III	Conditions for which there is evidence and/or general agreement that the procedure or treatment is not useful/effective and in some cases may be harmful.	
<u>Therapeutic recommendations</u>		
Level of Evidence A	Data derived from multiple randomized clinical trials or metaanalyses	
Level of Evidence B	Data derived from a single randomized trial or nonrandomized studies	
Level of Evidence C	Consensus opinion of experts, case studies, or standard of care	
<u>Diagnostic recommendations</u>		
Level of Evidence A	Data derived from multiple prospective cohort studies using a reference standard applied by a masked evaluator	
Level of Evidence B	Data derived from a single grade A study, or one or more case-control studies, or studies using a reference standard applied by an unmasked evaluator	
Level of Evidence C	Consensus opinion of experts	

Recommendations for BP (showed in Table1-3) (Hemphill, Greenberg et al. 2015):

1. For ICH patients presenting with SBP between 150 and 220 mmHg and without contraindication to acute BP treatment, acute lowering of SBP to 140 mmHg is safe (Class I; Level of Evidence A) and can be effective for improving functional outcome (Class IIa; Level of Evidence B). (Revised from the previous guideline)
2. For ICH patients presenting with SBP >220 mmHg, it may be reasonable to consider aggressive reduction of BP with a continuous intravenous infusion and frequent BP monitoring (Class IIb; Level of Evidence C). (New recommendation) (Hemphill, Greenberg et al. 2015).

4.2.2. Serum Glucose Regulation

Hyperglycemia on admission has been associated with poor outcome after intracerebral hemorrhage. However, the mechanistic links between hyperglycemia and hematoma expansion are not fully elucidated.

Table 3. Class I Recommendations for management of ICH

Section	Class I recommendations
Emergency Diagnosis and Assessment	Perform a baseline severity score as part of the initial evaluation of patients with ICH (Class I; level of evidence B; new recommendation). Rapid neuroimaging with computed tomography or MRI is recommended to distinguish ischemic stroke from ICH (Class I; level of evidence A; unchanged from the previous guideline).
Hemostasis and Coagulopathy, Antiplatelet Agents, and Deep-Vein Thrombosis Prophylaxis	Patients with a severe coagulation factor deficiency or severe thrombocytopenia should receive appropriate factor replacement therapy or platelets, respectively (Class I; level of evidence C; unchanged from the previous guideline). Patients with ICH whose international normalized ratio (INR) is elevated because of vitamin K antagonists (VKAs) should have their VKA withheld, receive therapy to replace vitamin K–dependent factors and correct the INR, and receive intravenous vitamin K (Class I; level of evidence C; unchanged from the previous guideline). Patients with ICH should have intermittent pneumatic compression for prevention of venous thromboembolism beginning the day of hospital admission (Class I; level of evidence A; revised from the previous guideline).
Blood Pressure	For patients with ICH presenting with systolic blood pressure (SBP) between 150 and 220 mm Hg and without contraindication to acute BP treatment, acute lowering of SBP to 140 mm Hg is safe (Class I; level of evidence A) and can be effective for improving functional outcome (Class IIa; level of evidence B; revised from the previous guideline)
General Monitoring and Nursing Care	Initial monitoring and management of patients with ICH should take place in an intensive care unit or dedicated stroke unit with physician and nursing neuroscience acute care expertise (Class I; level of evidence B; revised from the previous guideline).
Glucose Management	Glucose should be monitored. Both hyperglycemia and hypoglycemia should be avoided (Class I; level of evidence C; revised from the previous guideline).
Seizures and Antiseizure Drugs	Clinical seizures should be treated with antiseizure drugs (Class I; level of evidence A; unchanged from the previous guideline). Patients with a change in mental status who are found to have electrographic seizures on electroencephalography should be treated with antiseizure drugs (Class I; level of evidence C; unchanged from the previous guideline).
Management of Medical Complications	A formal screening procedure for dysphagia should be performed in all patients before the initiation of oral intake to reduce the risk for pneumonia (Class I; level of evidence B; new recommendation).
Surgical Treatment of ICH	Patients with cerebellar hemorrhage who are deteriorating neurologically or who have brainstem compression and/or hydrocephalus from ventricular obstruction should undergo surgical removal of the hemorrhage as soon as possible (Class I; level of evidence B; unchanged from the previous guideline).
Prevention of Recurrent ICH	BP should be controlled in all patients with ICH (Class I; level of evidence A; revised from the previous guideline); measures to control BP should begin immediately after ICH onset (Class I; level of evidence A; new recommendation).
Rehabilitation and Recovery	Given the potentially serious nature and complex pattern of evolving disability and the increasing evidence for efficacy, it is recommended that all patients with ICH have access to multidisciplinary rehabilitation (Class I; level of evidence A; revised from the previous guideline).

Serum glucose reduction is another possible clinical intervention. Although high levels of fasting plasma glucose may represent stress hyperglycemia caused by large hematomas or dense neurological deficits (Kazui, Minematsu et al. 1997, Ovesen, Havsteen et al. 2014), HbA1c would provide an estimate of control of diabetes mellitus or blood glucose level for the preceding three month period (Kazui, Minematsu et al. 1997). In addition to aggravating atherosclerosis and arteriolosclerosis (Kazui, Minematsu et al. 1997, Waje-Andreassen, Naess et al. 2015), hyperglycemia may precipitate hemorrhage expansion by the analogy with hemorrhagic infarction (Kazui, Minematsu et al. 1997). However an adverse result showed that high glucose was not associated with hematoma expansion (Feng, Tauhid et al. 2012). Some studies have reported evidence of hematoma growth from bleeding into an ischemic penumbra zone surrounding the hematoma, while other reports have not confirmed the existence of ischemia at the hypoperfused area in the periphery of the hematoma (Rincon and Mayer 2008, Rincon and Mayer 2012, Li, Fan et al. 2015). Decline in serum glucose concentration associated with a decrease in the proportion of subjects with hematoma expansion and poor clinical outcome (Qureshi, Palesch et al. 2011). The results provide a standard for a randomized, controlled clinical trial to evaluate the efficacy of aggressive serum glucose reduction in lessening mortality and disability among patients with ICH (Qureshi, Palesch et al. 2011).

High blood glucose on admission predicts an increased risk of mortality and poor outcome in patients with ICH, independent of the presence of diabetes mellitus. A randomized trial showing improved outcomes with tight glucose control (range, 80–110 mg/dL) using insulin infusions in mainly surgical critical care patients has increased the use of this therapy. However, more recent studies have demonstrated an increased incidence of systemic and cerebral hypoglycemic events and possibly even an increased risk of mortality in patients treated with this regimen. A cluster randomized trial of a set of interventions (managing glucose, fever, and swallowing dysfunction in stroke units) found improved outcomes in a mixed cohort of ischemic and hemorrhagic stroke patients. At present, the optimal management of hyperglycemia in ICH and the target glucose level remains to be clarified. Hypoglycemia should be avoided (Hemphill, Greenberg et al. 2015). Recommendation for Glucose Management:

Glucose should be monitored. Both hyperglycemia and hypoglycemia should be avoided (Class I; Level of Evidence C). (Revised from the previous guideline) (Hemphill, Greenberg et al. 2015).

4.2.3. Hemostatic Therapies

There is a systemic activation of hemostasis after acute ICH. However, most of thc changes in hemostatic protein levels were common to patients with or without hematoma expansion, and only the activity of factor XIII increased in those with hematoma expansion (Marti-Fabregas, Borrell et al. 2010). The investigators interpreted that patients with higher factor XIII activity were able to have faster and/or better-stabilized clots with enhanced resistance to endogenous lysis. Because of this increased utilization of factor XIII, its activity in peripheral blood decreased with time, whereas it was stable or increased in hematoma expansion patients (Marti-Fabregas, Borrell et al. 2010). It is possible that the increased activity of factor XIII possibly reflects the potentiated hemostasis to prevent the hematoma expansion and works as a self-compensatory or self-protective mechanism. As such, it is not advisable to intervene aggressively in the activity of factor XIII.

Fibrinogen is cross-linked with each other in the presence of factor XIII to become fibrin polymers, which are the final products of the coagulation cascade (the secondary hemostasis). Fibrinogen also takes part in primary hemostasis, i.e., platelet aggregation. Fibrinogen levels may represent the function of both blood coagulation and platelet aggregation (Fujii, Takeuchi et al. 1998). Fibrinogen is a critical protein for hemostasis and clot formation. Fibrinogen concentrates or cryoprecipitate (containing fibrinogen, factor VIII, von Willebrand factor, and FXIII) are more effective at fibrinogen repletion than transfusing plasma (Collis and Collins 2015, Levy and Goodnough 2015). Furthermore, rapid administration of antifibrinolytic, intravenous administration of 2g tranexamic acid over a period of 10 minutes, was recommended for prevention of hematoma growth in patients with ICH (Sorimachi, Fujii et al. 2005, Meretoja, Churilov et al. 2014).

International normalized ratio (INR) is the marker of coagulation. Impaired coagulation can potentially facilitate hematoma expansion (Emiru, Bershad et al. 2013), so its rapid reversal should be one of the main targets for this condition. The hemostatic impairment may be due to the intake of anticoagulants, antiplatelet agents, or inherited or acquired abnormalities in the coagulation system (Emiru, Bershad et al. 2013). The first consideration for emergency management of anticoagulant and antiplatelet-related hematoma expansion is to stop taking these agents. Correcting the INR to 1.3 or less within 2-4 hours has been shown to decrease hematoma expansion (Turpie 2008, Rincon and Mayer 2012, Kuramatsu, Gerner et al. 2015). Rapid reversal of coagulopathy is desirable to prevent ICH expansion. The most promising agents for rapid INR reversal to prevent hematoma expansion include recombinant activated factor VIIa (rFVIIa), fresh frozen plasma (FFP), intravenous vitamin K, and activated and inactivated prothrombin complex concentrates (PCCs) (Turpie 2008, Cairns, Connolly et al. 2011, Zhou, Schwarting et al. 2011, Emiru, Bershad et al. 2013, James, Palys et al. 2013, Zhou, Zorn et al. 2013, Yaghi, Eisenberger et al. 2014, Waje-Andreassen, Naess et al. 2015). Recombinant factor VIIa is effective for immediate INR reversal and prevention of hematoma expansion, but is also associated with increased thrombotic complications such as myocardial infarction, pulmonary embolism, and deep venous thrombosis (DVT). Recombinant factor VIIa has not been shown to improve survival or functional outcome and is generally not recommended for reversal in anticoagulant-related ICH (Rincon and Mayer 2012, Emiru, Bershad et al. 2013, James, Palys et al. 2013). Frozen plasma should only be used to reverse the warfarin effect when there is severe bleeding or hemostasis is required for emergent surgery or an invasive procedure (Tran, Chunilal et al. 2014). Frozen plasma should not be used as the first-line therapy for reversal of the warfarin effect except in severe urgent clinical situations, such as life-threatening hemorrhage (e.g., intracranial hemorrhage) and when prothrombin complex concentrate is not available (Baker, Coughlin et al. 2004, Zareh, Davis et al. 2011). FFP always requires large volume infusion and a slow thawing time, and can lead to transfusion-related complications such as infections, pulmonary edema and delayed reversal of INR (O'Shaughnessy, Atterbury et al. 2004, Turpie 2008, Cairns, Connolly et al. 2011, James, Palys et al. 2013). Vitamin K is essential but does not have a rapid effect, often taking 24 hours for INR reversal (Cairns, Connolly et al. 2011). PCCs are increasing in popularity as low-volume, rapid-reversal agents and have been reported to be superior to FFP and vitamin K in several studies (Yasaka, Oomura et al. 2003, van Aart, Eijkhout et al. 2006, Pabinger, Brenner et al. 2008, Kuramatsu, Huttner et al. 2013). Individualized dosing of PCC may be the most effective method of reversal. In one study, individualized dosing of PCC based on the patient's body weight and initial INR was superior at reaching the target INR 15 minutes after dosing compared with the standard dosage of PCC (van Aart, Eijkhout et al. 2006). Similar data has led to support for PCC as the standard of care at many institutions (Hanger, Geddes et al. 2013, James, Palys et al. 2013, Kuramatsu, Huttner et al. 2013). However, increasing concentrations of PPC can carry a risk of thromboembolic complications and disseminated intravascular coagulation (Kuramatsu, Huttner et al. 2013). As such, the optimal dosing and infusion rates of PCC to rapidly but safely reverse INR are not clearly defined.

Another possible strategy for reducing hematoma growth is to reverse the effect of antiplatelet medications by administering a platelet transfusion (Naidech, Jovanovic et al. 2009, Beshay, Morgan et al. 2010). Transfusion of 10–12.5 units of platelets has been shown to restore normal platelet function in patients on aspirin and clopidogrel (Vilahur, Choi et al. 2007). Desmopressin (0.4 μg/kg IV) has been known to improve platelet reactivity in patients treated with aspirin by releasing a greater number of von Willibrand multimers (Naidech, Maas et al. 2014).

Various hemostatic therapies have been considered for use in spontaneous intracranial hemorrhage. However, most of these have not been tested in larger clinical trials so far. In particular, rFVIIa seemed to be a promising candidate. In the Phase 2b trial that included 399 patients, we demonstrated treatment to significantly restrict hematoma expansion, improve functional outcome, and reduce mortality despite the fact that significantly more arterial thromboembolic events occurred in the group with the highest dose of 160 μg/kg. The Phase III trial FAST (Factor seven for Acute hemorrhagic Stroke Trial) included 816 patients who did either receive 20 or 80 μg/kg of rFVIIa or placebo. This trial confirmed the HE-restrictive properties of rFVIIa. However, this had no clinical effect either on functional outcome or on mortality. In a post hoc analysis, we found that limiting the trial population to patients with intracerebral hemorrhage volume <60 mL, with <5 mL of intraventricular hemorrhage, of an age <70 years and treatment within 2.5 hours to reveal positive clinical outcome not only in the FAST, but also in the Phase 2b data set. Another explanation for failure to prove clinical efficacy may be the fact that the pure difference in hematoma expansion restriction between treatment groups was simply too small to translate into a relevant clinical effect. These differences in hematoma volume range between 2 and 5 mL in rVFIIa-ICH-2b and FAST, comparable to trials on different treatments such as INTERACT and CHANT (Cerebral Hematoma and NXY Treatment trial; see subsequently) that equally failed to show an outcome benefit. Furthermore, there may be an upper threshold of absolute hematoma volume beyond which clinical improvement is not very likely, suggested to be above 60 to 80 mL. These results call for another trial on rFVIIa with stricter selection criteria of inclusion time window, intracerebral hemorrhage (and intraventricular hemorrhage) volume, and age of patients (Steiner and Bosel 2010).

Recommendations for hemostasis and coagulopathy, antiplatelet agents, and DVT prophylaxis (Hemphill, Greenberg et al. 2015) (see Table1-3):

1. Patients with a severe coagulation factor deficiency or severe thrombocytopenia should receive appropriate factor replacement therapy or platelets, respectively (Class I; Level of Evidence C). (Unchanged from the previous guideline)
2. Patients with ICH whose INR is elevated because of VKA should have their VKA withheld, receive therapy to replace vitamin K–dependent factors and correct the INR, and receive intravenous vitamin K (Class I; Level of Evidence C). PCCs may have fewer complications and correct the INR more rapidly than FFP and might be considered over FFP (Class IIb; Level of Evidence B). rFVIIa does not replace all clotting factors, and although the INR may be lowered, clotting may not be restored in vivo; therefore, rFVIIa is not recommended for VKA reversal in ICH (Class III; Level of Evidence C). (Revised from the previous guideline)
3. For patients with ICH who are taking dabigatran, rivaroxaban, or apixaban, treatment with FEIBA, other PCCs, or rFVIIa might be considered on an individual basis. Activated charcoal might be used if the most recent dose of dabigatran, apixaban, or rivaroxaban was taken.
4. Protamine sulfate may be considered to reverse heparin in patients with acute ICH (Class IIb; Level of Evidence C). (New recommendation)
5. The usefulness of platelet transfusions in ICH patients with a history of antiplatelet use is uncertain (Class IIb; Level of Evidence C). (Revised from the previous guideline)
6. Although rFVIIa can limit the extent of hematoma expansion in noncoagulopathic ICH patients, there is an increase in thromboembolic risk with rFVIIa and no clear clinical benefit in unselected patients. Thus, rFVIIa is not recommended (Class III; Level of Evidence A). (Unchanged from the previous guideline)
7. Patients with ICH should have intermittent pneumatic compression for prevention of venous thromboembolism beginning the day of hospital admission (Class I; Level of Evidence A). Graduated compression stockings are not beneficial to reduce DVT or improve outcome (Class III; Level of Evidence A). (Revised from the previous guideline)
8. After documentation of cessation of bleeding, low dose subcutaneous low-molecular-weight heparin or unfractionated heparin may be considered for prevention of venous thromboembolism in patients

with lack of mobility after 1 to 4 days from onset (Class IIb; Level of Evidence B). (Unchanged from the previous guideline)

9. Systemic anticoagulation or IVC filter placement is probably indicated in ICH patients with symptomatic DVT or PE (Class IIa; Level of Evidence C). The decision between these 2 options should take into account several factors, including time from hemorrhage onset, hematoma stability, cause of hemorrhage, and overall patient condition (Class IIa; Level of Evidence C). (New recommendation).

4.2.4. Creatinine and Possible Intervention

Creatinine is a recognized marker of long-standing hypertension with accumulated vascular injury and increased fragility of small vessels. Elevated creatinine levels may reflect severe renal dysfunction, which is associated with impaired platelet function (Mannucci and Tripodi 2012) and uncontrolled hypertension or diabetes mellitus (Kazui, Minematsu et al. 1997). Additional factors may be accelerative of creatinine increases, such as patient hydration status and diabetes history. The monitoring of appropriate drug therapy, especially drugs which are cleared by the kidneys to prevent rise of serum creatinine, is more important than therapy for lowering creatinine. The adoption of maintenance dialysis was the first step that improved the bleeding tendency in uremia, although not fully satisfactorily (Mannucci and Tripodi 2012), and heparin administration could induce hematoma expansion (Emiru, Bershad et al. 2013, James, Palys et al. 2013).

The regular administration of erythropoietin has minimized the frequency and severity of bleeding symptoms in patients with end-stage renal insufficiency beyond the benefits obtained by dialysis (Mannucci and Tripodi 2012). In handling the management and prevention of spontaneous bleeding, some drugs have been found to shorten the prolonged bleeding time (i.e., desmopressin with a short-lasting effect and conjugated estrogens with a more prolonged effect) (Mannucci and Tripodi 2012). Because these medications cannot be administered prophylactically for prolonged periods of time, long-lasting prevention of the bleeding tendency in uremia remains unsettled (Mannucci and Tripodi 2012).

4.2.5. Serum Cholesterol and Intervention

The role of serum cholesterol is to maintain the integrity of vascular vessels. Decreased low-density lipoprotein cholesterol (LDL-C) and total-C levels have been previously demonstrated to be associated with a higher risk of ICH. Moreover, both lower total-C and LDL-C levels have been shown to increase risk of death after ICH in several studies (Rodriguez-Luna, Rubiera et al. 2011). Lower cholesterol levels have been related to the development of medial smooth muscle cell necrosis (Ooneda, Yoshida et al. 1978, Rodriguez-Luna, Rubiera et al. 2011), thus decreasing the resistance to rupturing of the vascular wall. Moreover, cholesterol levels modify platelet aggregability by their action on the platelet activating factor, so that lower cholesterol levels may decrease platelet aggregation (Chui, Marotta et al. 1991), thus predisposing the individual to ICH growth (Rodriguez-Luna, Rubiera et al. 2011). LDL-C levels were inversely correlated and independently associated with hematoma expansion at 24 hours. Moreover, lower LDL-C levels (<95 mg/dL) independently predicted early neurological deterioration and 3-month mortality. However, LDL-C was unrelated to poor long-term outcome after acute ICH (Rodriguez-Luna, Rubiera et al. 2011).

However, no relationship was found between lipid-lowering agents and hematoma expansion (Rodriguez-Luna, Rubiera et al. 2011, Priglinger, Arima et al. 2015). Higher intake of saturated fat, which leads to higher LDL cholesterol concentrations, was shown to be associated with reduced risk of intraparenchymal hemorrhage for both Japanese and American patients (Iso, Sato et al. 2003, Noda, Iso et al. 2009). A high fat diet may be beneficial to patients suffering from hematoma expansion.

5. New Molecular Predictors for Hematoma Expansion and Corresponding Intervention

5.1. Function and Inhibition of Plasma Kallikrein

The role of plasma kallikrein (PK) in cerebral hematoma expansion with hyperglycemia has been reported (Liu, Gao et al. 2011). Plasma kallikrein is activated during hemorrhage by the contact system and plays a key role in innate inflammation, vascular function, the intrinsic coagulation cascade, and the fibrinolytic system (Liu, Gao et al. 2010, Liu, Gao et al. 2011, Bjorkqvist, Jamsa et al. 2013). Hyperglycemia promotes ICH through PK-mediated inhibition of the platelet-vessel wall interaction. PK exerts potent anti-hemostatic function in diabetic rodent models, and this effect is greatly enhanced in hyperglycemic blood (Liu, Gao et al. 2010, Liu, Gao et al. 2011, Bjorkqvist, Jamsa et al. 2013). Adhesion of PK to collagens blocks binding sites for platelet glycoprotein VI receptors (GPVI) and inhibits platelet aggregation on collagen fibers at the injury site, leading to sustained bleeding and hematoma expansion (Liu, Gao et al. 2010, Liu, Gao ct al. 2011, Bjorkqvist, Jamsa et al. 2013). These findings suggest targeting PK for prevention of brain hematoma in hyperglycemic patients (Liu, Gao et al. 2010, Liu, Gao et al. 2011, Bjorkqvist, Jamsa et al. 2013). Further studies are required to verify this confusing hypothesis in animals and patients with ICH (Liu, Gao et al. 2010).

Systemic administration of a small molecule PK inhibitor, ASP-440 (Phipps, Clermont et al. 2009, Clermont, Chilcote et al. 2011), reduced hematoma expansion in DM rats (Liu, Gao et al. 2011), which is similar to the effects of PK-deficiency in humans (Asmis, Sulzer et al. 2002). Treatment of DM rats with ASP-440 increased aPTT and tail bleeding time, while reducing hematoma expansion induced by autologous blood. ASP-440 is believed to reduce hematoma expansion by suppressing the formation of PK from prekallikrein, possibly mediated by inhibition of the contact activation system (Liu, Gao et al. 2011). The mechanism for PK inhibition of collagen-induced platelet aggregation requires further experiments to confirm.

5.2. Von Willebrand Factor and Intervention

Von Willebrand factor (vWF) is a plasma protein that is involved in thrombosis and hemostasis (Sadler 1998, Arslan, Yoldas et al. 2013). VWF mediates the adhesion of platelets to sites of vascular injury and forms (Arslan, Yoldas et al. 2013) an adhesive bridge between platelets and vascular subendothelial structures, as well as between adjacent platelets at sides of endothelial injury (Arslan, Yoldas et al. 2013). Increased platelet aggregation and pathological thrombus formation strongly rely on endothelial vWF accumulation and plasma vWF adhesion (Li, Fan et al. 2015). Recent research results showed the role of vWF genetic variant in increasing risk for hematoma expansion after ICH (Appelboom, Piazza et al. 2013). This research suggested that vWF rs216321 SNP genotype independently predicted relative hematoma enlargement, even when controlling known risk factors for hematoma growth (Appelboom, Piazza et al. 2013), and confirmed the role of hemostatic polymorphism on hematoma expansion (Appelboom, Piazza et al. 2013). VWF dysfunction was thought to be an important culprit in bleeding disorders. A target therapy for vWF in hematoma expansion has been reported. Desmopressin is a vasopressin agonist used as first-line therapy for mild-to-moderate vWF deficiency or hemophilia (Mannucci, Ruggeri et al. 1977, Teng, Mitchell et al. 2014). Desmopressin is widely used in the management of bleeding disorders and improves primary hemostasis through up-regulation of plasma vWF and factor VIII, while having possible direct effects on platelet reactivity (Teng, Mitchell et al. 2014). Desmopressin leads to the release of vWF and reduces clinical bleeding (Naidech, Maas et al. 2014). Desmopressin improved platelet activity, increased vWF antigen levels, and hematoma expansion was muted in the subset of patients treated within 12 hours of ICH symptom onset (Naidech, Maas et al. 2014). Given its safety, low cost, and reduction in clinical bleeding, desmopressin is an attractive pharmacological treatment for acute ICH (Naidech, Maas et al. 2014). Cryoprecipitate (a plasma product rich in vWF) should be considered for patients with vWF genetic variation and/or patients unresponsive to desmopressin in hematoma expansion.

5.3. N-methyl-D-Aspartate (NMDA) and Its Receptor Antagonist

Overactivation of the extrasynaptic N-methyl-D-aspartate (NMDA)-type receptors is a major route for excessive Ca2+ influx in triggering excitotoxic neuronal cell damage or death (Lipton 2007, Song and Yu 2014). Glutamate stimulation of the metabotropic glutamate receptors leads to a vertiginous increase in neuronal tPA synthesis (Shin, Kundel et al. 2004). Some reports suggest that tPA cleaves the NR1 subunit of the NMDAR and strengthens NMDA toxicity via the magnification of NMDA calcium currents (Nicole, Docagne et al. 2001, Gravanis and Tsirka 2005). Thus, this cascade of reactions, which involves glutamate, NMDAR, and tPA, constitutes a vicious cycle which ends in catastrophic neurotoxicity (Liu, Cheng et al. 2004) (showed in Figure 1-3). Memantine, which is known to be a moderate-affinity, uncompetitive NMDA receptor antagonist, was found to reduce hemorrhagic extension and to exert a complicated inhibitory effect on glutamate overstimulation, tissue plasminogen activator (tPA) upregulation, and matrix metalloproteinase (MMP)-9 increment in hemorrhagic rat brains (Lee, Chu et al. 2006). Memantine (20 mg/kg/day) was intraperitoneally administered 30 min after the induction of ICH, and at daily intervals afterwards, for either 3 or 14 days (Lee, Chu et al. 2006). The mechanisms underlying NMDA's association with hematoma expansion are not fully understood but warrant further consideration.

5.4. Inflammatory Markers and Possible Intervention

Inflammatory responses participate in the pathophysiological processes of brain injury following ICH (Chen, Yang et al. 2015). They can result in disruption of the blood–brain barrier, elicit brain edema, and contribute to cell death after hemorrhage via cytotoxic mediators (Du, Yang et al. 2013, Gu, Xuan et al. 2013, Di Napoli, Parry-Jones et al. 2014, Chen, Yang et al. 2015). Activation of innate immunity and inflammatory responses also contributes to progression of brain edema and hematoma expansion after ICH (Figure 1-4) (Silva, Leira et al. 2005, Mingam, Moranis et al. 2008, Osuka, Watanabe et al. 2013, Hunter and Jones 2015, Wang and Zhang 2016).

Interleukin-6 (IL-6) represents a keystone cytokine in infection, cancer and inflammation, in which it speeds up disease progression or supports the maintenance of immunological reactions (Grivennikov and Karin 2010). IL-6 can induce amplification of gap junctions of endothelial cells and enlarge vascular permeability by altering actin filaments and by transforming the shape of endothelial cells (Osuka, Watanabe et al. 2013, Gonzalez-Moreno, Camara-Lemarroy et al. 2014). Binding of IL-6 to its receptor induces the phosphorylation of receptor-associated Janus kinases (JAK), allowing the recruitment of signal transducer and activator of transcription STAT1 and STAT3 (Mingam, Moranis et al. 2008, Di Napoli, Godoy et al. 2012). STAT3 can bind to NF-κB then facilitate NF- κ B activation and nuclear entry (Yao, Zhu et al. 2011, Huang, Dai et al. 2013). NF-κB, known to stimulate inflammatory cytokine production, inflammatory cell function, and endothelial injury, ultimately caused increased injury (Kim, Ryu et al. 2013) after ICH. One study showed that IL-6 levels >24 pg/mL increased 16-fold the risk of early hematoma expansion after controlling for other markers of inflammation (Silva, Leira et al. 2005). Tocilizumab, which targets the receptor for IL-6 (IL-6R) in the treatment of inflammatory arthritis and a subset of other immunological conditions, has been identified (Grivennikov and Karin 2010) as an effective intervention. Tocilizumab may exert possible protective effects on hematoma expansion and block this vicious cycle, but there are no reports as yet on its efficacy in treating ICH.

C-reactive protein (CRP), an acute-phase reactant induced by IL-6, was associated with hematoma expansion as well as IL-6 in ICH patients [108]. One study demonstrated that plasma CRP>10 mg/L within the first few hours of spontaneous ICH was independently predictive of both early hematoma expansion and early neurological worsening, both of which are associated with increased mortality (Hunter and Jones 2015). It is likely that both inflammatory factors impair coagulation function and vessel wall pathophysiology and contribute to a persistent vessel leak (Nandi, Tahiliani et al. 2006, Hunter and Jones 2015).

Visfatin is a novel adipokine with different functions. Visfatin can accelerate up -regulation of inflammatory cytokines and chemokines and has a link with a proinflammatory state that may contribute to poor clinical outcomes after acute ICH (Sinn, Lee et al. 2007, Gu, Xuan et al. 2013). Visfatin is also released by IL-6 in cells involving innate immunity (Huang, Dai et al. 2013), and plasma visfatin level was highly correlated with plasma CRP (Sinn, Lee et al. 2007, Mingam, Moranis et al. 2008, Gu, Xuan et al. 2013). Visfatin has been demonstrated to positively correlate with ICH severity and inflammatory biomarkers such as CRP and also hematoma expansion at 24 hours, supporting an inflammatory role of visfatin in progression of hematoma expansion after ICH (Mingam, Moranis et al. 2008).

Leptin, another important adipokine, is not only an energy regulator but also a novel mediator of inflammation (Kim, Ryu et al. 2013). Leptin promotes phagocytosis by monocytes/ macrophages and their secretion of proinflammatory cytokines (Kim, Ryu et al. 2013) such as IL-6 and tumor necrosis factor- α (TNF-α) (Gong, Ennis et al. 2001). This detrimental effect of leptin on ICH is mediated by the STAT3 signaling pathway in inflammatory cells (Gong, Ennis et al. 2001). As previously mentioned, a connection between STAT3 and hematoma expansion has been demonstrated (Huang, Dai et al. 2013). Similarly to visfatin, Plasma leptin levels were positively correlated and independently associated with hematoma expansion, ICH severity, and CRP (Sinn, Lee et al. 2007, Du, Yang et al. 2013, Osuka, Watanabe et al. 2013).

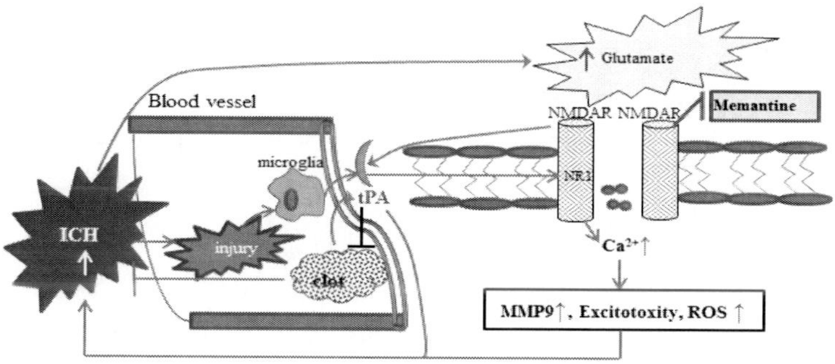

Figure 5. Schematic pathway of N-methyl-D-aspartate receptor (NMDAR) in hematoma expansion.

The ubiquitin-proteasome system (UPS) regulates inflammatory response via the up-regulation of several pro-inflammatory molecules (NF-κB and IL-6) (Keynes and Garthwaite 2004, Sinn, Lee et al. 2007). The relation of IL-6, NF-κB and hematoma expansion has been discussed previously (Kim, Ryu et al. 2013, Gonzalez-Moreno, Camara-Lemarroy et al. 2014). Bortezomib, a proteasome inhibitor, has anti-inflammatory effects in reducing both hematoma expansion and brain edema during the early period of ICH (Makogonenko, Tsurupa et al. 2002). The mechanism of proteasome inhibition was thought to be associated with the reduction of COX2 and iNOS after ICH, resulting in the attenuation of vasodilation and perturbing the integrity of the vascular barrier induced by COX2 (Makogonenko, Tsurupa et al. 2002, Sinn, Lee et al. 2007, Ho-Tin-Noe, Demers et al. 2011), also protecting against oxidative injury, abnormal mitochondrial respiration and DNA damage induced by iNOS (Lei, Mace et al. 2012). A single intravenous 0.2 mg/kg dose of bortezomib inhibited the early hematoma growth occurring within 24 hours and diminished hematoma volume after 72 hours (Makogonenko, Tsurupa et al. 2002). Because bortezomib is now used in human treatment, with few side effects, its therapeutic application for ICH seems available, although its precise mechanism and validity in inhibiting hematoma growth after ICH requires further confirmation.

The signaling cassette that controls the activity of IL-6/ CRP/visfatin/leptin is complicated (showed in Figure 6)(Wang and Zhang 2016), and more research on the underlying mechanism is required to determine potential intervention strategies.

5.5. Molecular Vascular Injury and Hematoma Expansion

5.5.1. Cellular Fibronectin

Cellular fibronectin (c-Fn), as a basal membrane component, is a glycoprotein especially important for the adhesion of platelets to fibrin, a function necessary for the blockage of bleeding (Biffi, Sonni et al. 2010). One research study demonstrated that plasma c-Fn levels >6 μg/mL were associated with a 92 -fold increase in the risk of early hematoma expansion, and c-Fn levels showed a high correlation with the percentage of the ICH growth. This study suggested c-Fn was the most powerful predictor of ICH enlargement (Silva, Leira et al. 2005). C-Fn is largely confined to the vascular endothelium, and high plasma levels of C-Fn might be indicative of endothelial damage and loss of microvascular integrity (Silva, Leira et al.

2005). As c-Fn plays an key role in blood clot formation by mediating the adhesion of platelets to fibrin (Silva, Leira et al. 2005, Biffi, Sonni et al. 2010), the disappearance of c-Fn in the vascular endothelium might compromise this clotting mechanism and facilitate ICH expansion (Silva, Leira et al. 2005).

Plasma c-Fn is a marker of vascular injury, and there is no better way to intervene in this process except by preventing its occurrence and maintaining vascular integrity. Improving or modulating the function of platelet plug formation is a potential means to preserve the structural integrity of intact blood vessels (Brouwers, Biffi et al. 2012) in the future.

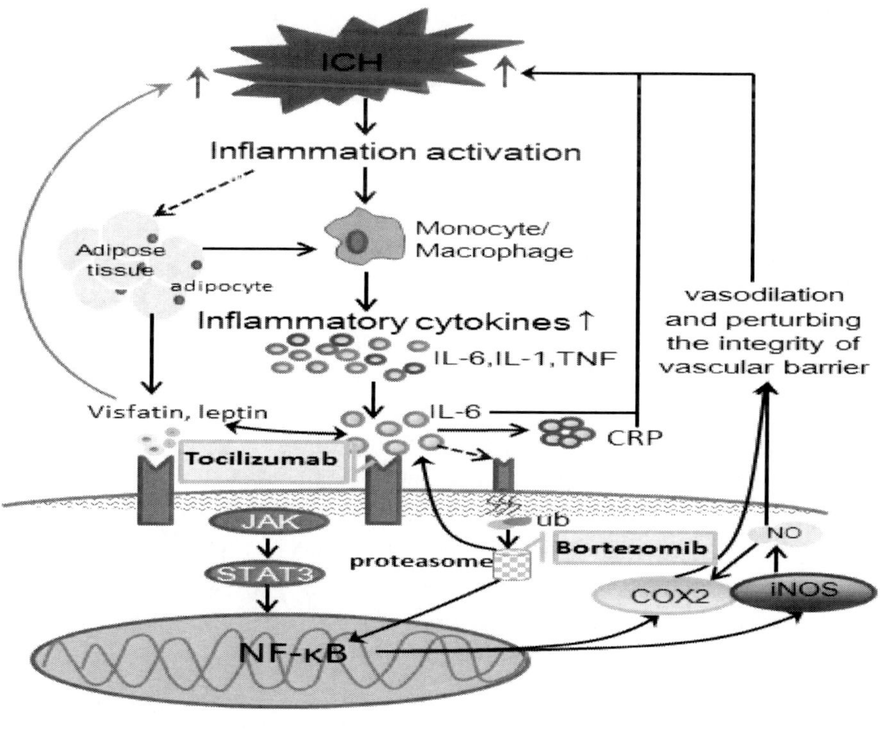

Figure 6. Schematic representation of various inflammatory cytokines and adipokines function on hematoma expansion.

5.5.2. Apolipoprotein Eε Alleles

Apolipoprotein E (APOE) ε2 and ε4 alleles are independent risk factors for spontaneous ICH in the lobar brain regions (Biffi, Sonni et al. 2010, Biffi, Anderson et al. 2011), most likely a reflection of their role in cerebral amyloid angiopathy (CAA) (Brouwers, Biffi et al. 2012, Rannikmae, Kalaria et al.

2014). The $\epsilon 4$ allele increases the severity of vascular amyloid deposition, whereas the $\epsilon 2$ allele appears to cause increased vasculopathic changes that lead to vessel rupture (Brouwers, Biffi et al. 2012, Rannikmae, Kalaria et al. 2014, Montanola, de Retana et al. 2016). A multicenter genetic association study showed that larger ICH volume is associated with the APOE $\epsilon 2$, but not $\epsilon 4$, allele. APOE $\epsilon 2$ carriers are at disproportionately increased risk of mortality and poor outcome after ICH (Brouwers, Biffi et al. 2012). One study demonstrated that the APOE $\epsilon 2$ allele is associated with hematoma expansion in patients with lobar ICH (Brouwers, Biffi et al. 2012, Chen, Zeng et al. 2014, Rannikmae, Kalaria et al. 2014).

There are no available interventions for the APOE $\epsilon 2$ allele, but APOE $\epsilon 2$ allele knock-out may be introduced into animal experiment protocols in the next few years.

CHALLENGES AND FUTURE DIRECTIONS

Hematoma expansion is an attractive endpoint for clinical trials, because of its correlation with outcome and the potential to intervene to prevent its occurrence. Substantial challenges remain, however, which will need to be addressed before successful translation to clinical outcomes (Brouwers and Greenberg 2013).

One major challenge will be to identify conditions under which preventing hematoma expansion actually improves clinical outcome. This point is underlined by the observation that although both rFVIIa trials found that hematoma expansion could be reduced, functional outcome in the phase III trial was not improved (Mayer, Brun et al. 2008). As it seems unlikely that hematoma expansion is clinically meaningless, the more plausible explanation is that the benefits of reducing expansion may have been outweighed by the thromboembolic risks of rFVIIa, particularly in those subjects who would not have expanded even without active treatment. By this reasoning, therapies that carry risk as well as benefit may need to be focused on selected patients at highest risk for subsequent hematoma expansion.

This consideration raises the second challenge of identifying more reliable predictors of hematoma expansion. Early presentation (within 4 – 6 hours) was used in the blood pressure reduction and rFVIIa trials as a surrogate for expansion, but only up to 40% of those patients actually suffer significant hematoma expansion (Brott, Broderick et al. 1997). The CTA spot sign was found to have a higher positive predictive value of 61% in a recent prospective study, and might therefore be a better (although still imperfect) predictor of expansion (Brouwers, Goldstein et al. 2012, Demchuk, Dowlatshahi et al. 2012). Identifying more accurate predictors of hematoma expansion thus remains a key research priority (Brouwers and Greenberg 2013).

A third challenge is that those patients at highest risk for expansion may have poor outcomes even if expansion is fully prevented. This concern is raised by the observation that the main risk factors for hematoma expansion, such as baseline ICH volume and anticoagulation use, also independently worsen ICH outcome. Our poor ability to reverse these accompanying factors might be indeed another reason behind the negative results of the phase III rFVIIa trial (Brouwers and Greenberg 2013).

This consideration raises the possibility that treatments that go beyond preventing expansion, potentially including surgical hematoma evacuation (as currently tested in the STICH II trial) or neuroprotective agents to salvage damaged brain tissue (such as deferoxamine), may be required for demonstrably improved ICH outcome (Brouwers and Greenberg 2013).

A final important consideration regarding hematoma expansion is the window it provides on the broader process of ICH pathogenesis. The expansion that can be measured after clinical presentation presumably represents only the tail end of an event that began with the first rupture of a diseased small vessel and progressively grew into a symptomatic macrobleed. Understanding the mechanisms that underlie this process, such as the secondary rupture of adjacent vessels described above, has the potential to lead not only to acute treatments for use after presentation, but also to novel preventive strategies for keeping small vessel ruptures from evolving into symptomatic macroscopic events (Brouwers and Greenberg 2013).

Although these major challenges are still unsolved, substantial progress has been made over the last decades to better understand and potentially treat hematoma expansion. Hematoma expansion remains the most readily modifiable marker of outcome, and thus a promising therapeutic target for intracerebral hemorrhage.

Conclusion

Taking together, most studies of hematoma expansion were in the clinical environment where intervention was difficult. However, there remain some indexes that should be considered for prevention and treatment. In this part, available information from clinical signs to molecular mechanisms is provided and potential intervention strategies discussed (Figure 7) (Wang and Zhang 2016). Prospective study for hematoma expansion and how to predict the paticnts who are at highest risk of hematoma expansion is more challengeable than restricting hematoma expansion itself following acute ICH.

So seeking and detecting risk markers in plasma that can be intervened appropriately is meaningful for patients with potential hematoma expansion, which may contribute to improve clinical outcomes in patients suffering from ICH.

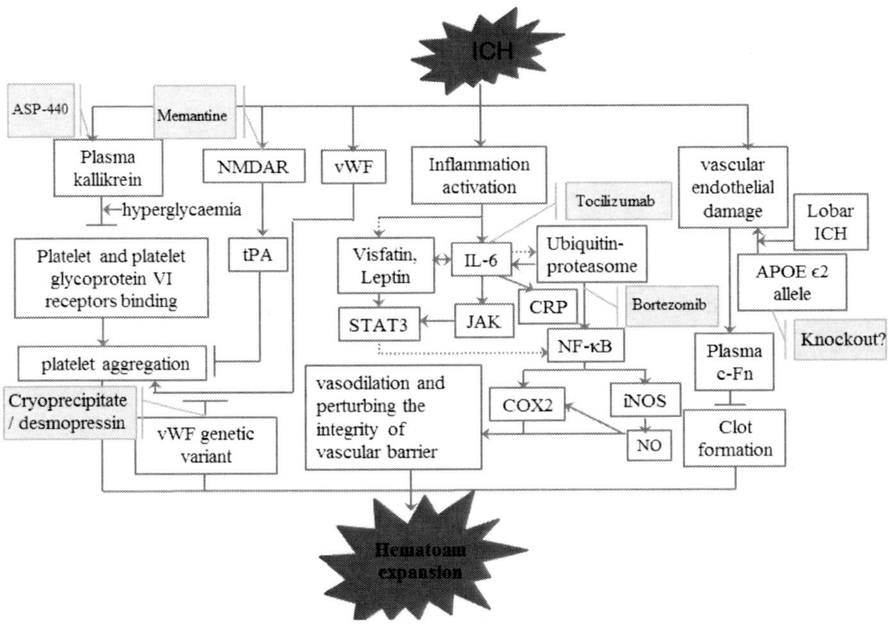

Figure 7. Summary of current understanding from molecular pathways and underlying intervention on hematoma expansion.

Chapter 3

HEMATOMA RESOLUTION IN INTRACEREBRAL HEMORRHAGE: FROM MECHANISMS TO CLINICAL TRANSLATION

ABSTRACT

Endogenous garbage cleaning system also known as scavenger receptors play important roles in the regulation of hematoma resolution in ICH. We try to illustrate how the endogenous hematoma scavenging system or scavenger receptors system in the brain work together to remove blood from the brain and reduce secondary brain insults, and presents potential clinically relevant molecular targets that could be harnessed to speed up this process via the endogenous phagocytosis. Meanwhile, guidelines of recommendations for clinical management of ICH are provided.

INTRODUCTION

Extravasated blood and subsequent intrahematoma hemolytic products trigger a series of adverse events after intracerebral hemorrhage (ICH), leading to secondary brain injury, edema and severe neurological deficits or death. Hematomas are the primary cause of neurologic deficits associated with ICH. Although the hematoma in human's brain gradually resolves within months, full restoration of neurological function can be slow and often incomplete, leaving survivors with devastating neurological deficits. Unless hematoma is cleared, the reservoirs of blood continue to inflict injury to neurovascular structures and blunt the brain repair processes (Zhao, Sun et al. 2015). However only a few evidence-based targeted treatments are used for ICH management, and interventions focus primarily on supportive care and comorbidity prevention. Effective hematoma removal and/or facilitating hematoma absorption result in the removal of all the toxic components, which is a goal and a novel therapeutic strategy for ICH, as hematoma removal/resolution can relieve mechanical compression, limit inflammatory injury, and promote the recovery of neuronal function (Zhao, Sun et al. 2007, Zhao, Grotta et al. 2009, Fang, Wang et al. 2013), although the mechanism of hematoma absorptions is unclear (Fang, Chen et al. 2014). Faster hematoma removal prevents secondary damage caused by the toxicity of the hematoma and hematoma-induced inflammation.

Endogenous garbage cleaning system also known as scavenger receptors play important roles in the regulation of hematoma resolution in ICH (Husemann, Loike et al. 2002). This review seeks to understand how the endogenous garbage-cleaning system or scavenger receptors system in the brain work together to remove blood from the brain and reduce brain damage, then find a medical measure to speed up this procedure.

1. Erythrolysis Following ICH

After an intracerebral hemorrhage, lysis of red blood cells (RBCs) in the hematoma results in brain edema formation, neuronal death and neurological deficits. A cascade of events triggered by erythrocyte lysis is critical for the secondary brain damage after ICH (Wang, Yang et al. 2011). The release of hemoglobin and its degradation products including iron from erythrocytes are involved in brain injury following ICH (Guo, Hua et al. 2012). Brain edema formation following ICH appears to be partly related to erythrocyte lysis and hemoglobin release (Qing, Dong et al. 2009). Oxidative stress caused by components of the lysed erythrocytes contributes to the brain injury after ICH (Wu, Hua et al. 2002).

Therefore, finding means of controlling hemolysis, and detoxification, and absorption of Hb, heme and iron may have important clinical implications. The removal of the hematoma and its blood components may be a key strategy to ameliorating the brain injury and improving recovery following ICH (Wang, Manaenko et al. 2016).

No effective therapy is available for treating ICH. One of several key components of brain damage after ICH is the neurotoxicity of blood products. Within hours to days after ICH, extravasated erythrocytes in the hematoma undergo lysis, releasing cytotoxic hemoglobin, heme, and iron, thereby initiating secondary processes, which negatively influence the viability of cells surrounding the hematoma. To offset this process, phagocytic cells, including the brain's microglia and hematogenous macrophages, phagocytose and then process extravasated erythrocytes before lysis and subsequent toxicity occurs (Zhao, Grotta et al. 2009). So the better understanding of phagocytosis through corresponding scavenger receptors is beneficial to explore removal of blood from the ICH-affected brain, thus limiting/preventing hemolysis from occurring. Scavenger receptors play important roles in the regulation of phagocytosis in macrophages (Husemann, Loike et al. 2002). The potential endogenous scavenger receptors/hematoma scavenging system following ICH were enumerated in Figure 8.

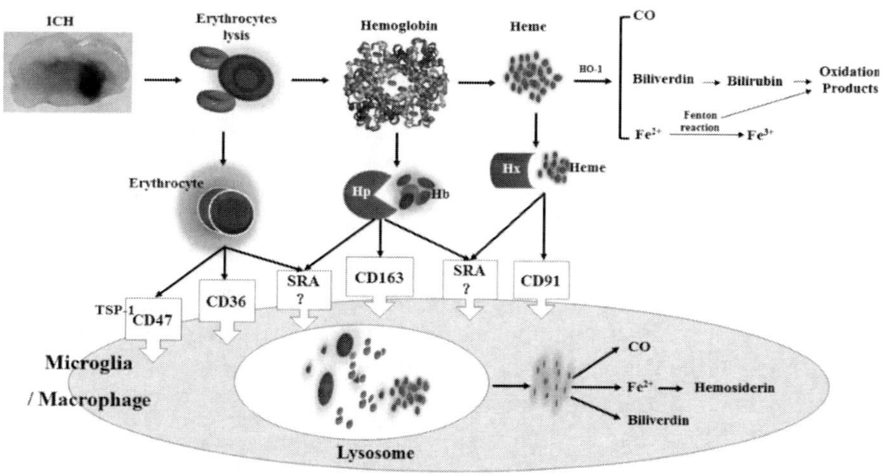

Figure 8. The graphic of potential endogenous hematoma scavenging system following ICH.

2. Phagocytosis in Hematoma Resolution

After ICH, phagocytosis-mediated clearance of apoptotic or damaged cells and dislocated blood components by macrophages (MMΦ) is believed to play a beneficial role by minimizing the exposure of the brain tissue to this toxic and pro-inflammatory milieu (Zhao, Gonzales et al. 2015). Phagocytosis is necessary to eliminate the hematoma after ICH. Microglia/ MMΦ represent the primary phagocytic system and the first line of defense against brain injuries that mediates the cleanup of hematoma. Thus, the efficacy of phagocytic function by Microglia/MMΦ is an essential step in limiting ICH-mediated damage (Zhao, Sun et al. 2015). The resident microglia and peripheral macrophages are rapidly mobilized to the lesions and initiate the release of mediators and recruitment of other immune cells (Schilling, Besselmann et al. 2005). Microglia is a key factor to remove the hematoma and clear debris, but it is a source of ongoing inflammation. Activated Microglia/MMΦ may trigger different function in response to specific situation just like a double-edged sword. The activation have dual effects on brain, it may play a potentially detrimental neurotoxic role by eliciting the expression of pro-inflammatory and initiating neuroprotective properties (Hu, Li et al. 2012, Wang, Tan et al. 2015). Although overactivation of microglia/ MMΦ amplifies inflammatory neuronal damage and represents a promising target for stroke management, anti-inflammatory agents have failed to show clinical benefits in many stroke trials so far (Hu, Li et al. 2012, Xing, Arai et al. 2012). The undesired effects may result from a broad suppression of microglia/ MMΦ which deprive the normal defensive functions of brain. It is worth noting that acute inflammation serves many protective functions, whereas chronic inflammation is more likely to exacerbate injury. So experimental stroke therapies should be shifted from blanketed microglia/ MMΦ suppression toward a more nuanced adjustment of the balance between protective and toxic microglia/MMΦ phenotypes (Hu, Li et al. 2012). Phagocyte activation inevitably release proinflammatory mediators and free radicals during hematoma resolution is toxic to neighboring cells, leading to secondary brain injury, but promotion of phagocytosis in a timely and efficient manner may limit the toxic effects of persistent blood products on surrounding tissue and may be important for recovery after ICH (Zhao, Sun et al. 2007). The process of the hematoma resolution probably be related to the concomitant acute brain swelling (Servadei, Staffa et al. 1989). So targeted stimulation of phagocytosis to promote efficient removal of the hematoma without/lessening harming surrounding brain cells may be a therapeutic option for ICH (Gonzales, Shah et al. 2013). Scavenger receptors, expressed on microglia/astrocytes or endothelia cells, play important roles in the regulation of phagocytosis in microglia/MMΦ (Doens and Fernandez 2014). Recent studies found that enhancing microglia/macrophage-mediated phagocytosis speeds up hematoma clearance then improves functional outcome after ICH (Zhao, Sun et al. 2015).

Microglia/Macrophages (MMΦ) utilize the scavenger receptors to participate in hematoma cleanup process after intracerebral hemorrhage.

3. Potential Endogenous Hematoma Scavenger Receptors after ICH

Hematomas are the primary cause of neurologic deficits associated with ICH. The early stages of hematoma compression cause deformation and mechanical injury to local brain tissues. Secondary neuronal damage is caused by direct toxicity and inflammatory responses induced by the components and metabolic products of late-stage hematomas and aggravates neurologic deficits (Keep, Hua et al. 2012). Therefore, effective hematoma removal is a goal of ICH treatment, as hematoma removal can relieve mechanical compression, limit inflammatory injury, and promote the recovery of neuronal function (Zhao, Sun et al. 2007). Clinically, the rate of hematoma absorption in patients with ICH correlates with the degree of neurologic deficit (Fang, Chen et al. 2014).

Scavenger receptors play important roles in the regulation of phagocytosis in macrophages. Scavenger receptor class A (SR-A, CD204), scavenger receptor-BI (SR-BI), and CD36 are cell surface proteins that mediate cell adhesion to, and endocytosis of, various native and pathologically modified substances, and participate in intracellular signaling, lipid metabolism, and host defense against bacterial pathogens. Microglia, Mato cells, astrocytes, cerebral microvascular endothelial cells, cerebral arterial smooth muscle cells, and retinal pigment epithelial cells express one or more of these scavenger receptors (Husemann, Loike et al. 2002).

3.1. CD36

CD36 is a well-recognized integral microglia/macrophage cell membrane protein and a type II scavenger receptor that can bind to modified lipids, symmetric red cell ghosts, or apoptotic neutrophils; this receptor expressed on the surface of macrophages and monocytes and plays an important role in mediating the recognition and phagocytosis (Zhao, Grotta et al. 2009, Fang,

Chen et al. 2014, Lagasse, Anidi et al. 2015). Microglia/Macrophages (MMφ) utilize the scavenger receptor CD36 to internalize the red blood cells (RBC) during the hematoma cleanup process after intracerebral hemorrhage. CD36-mediated hematoma absorption occurs in ICH patients and that this absorption is significantly associated with patient prognosis. The results of in vitro and in vivo experiments related to ICH further confirmed that CD36 promotes hematoma absorption. After the onset of ICH, inflammatory factors induced by the activation of the TLR4 signaling pathway downregulate CD36 expression and inhibit hematoma absorption. The application of TLR4 inhibitors could upregulate CD36 expression and increase hematoma absorption. To our knowledge, our study is the first to clarify the mechanism underlying hematoma absorption in patients with ICH; the results of this study provide reliable experimental data that may contribute to the development of clinical treatments that promote hematoma absorption in patients with ICH. Activation of TLR4 signaling following ICH may have a negative regulatory effect on CD36 expression (Fang, Chen et al. 2014). Cells lacking phagocytic abilities acquire phagocytic functions following transfection with CD36. A peroxisome proliferator-activated receptor γ agonist promotes hematoma absorption following ICH, which significantly reduces secondary inflammatory damages; the mechanism may be associated with the upregulation of CD36 expression in the microglia. Cells lacking phagocytic abilities acquire phagocytic functions following transfection with CD36 (Cao, Luo et al. 2016). The low levels of CD36 present may control adhesion of erythrocytes and may have a signal transduction role in platelets and monocytes. CD36 and thrombospondin (TSP) appear to be involved in several cell adhesion processes, including thrombin-induced platelet aggregation, adhesion of platelets to monocytes and so on (van Schravendijk, Handunnetti et al. 1992). However, the function of CD36 and the regulatory mechanism underlying the effect of CD36 in hematoma absorption are unclear.

3.2. CD47

CD47 is an integrin-associated transmembrane protein expressed in a variety of cells types including microglia/ MMΦ, oliogodendrocytes and erythrocytes (Burger, de Korte et al. 2012, Zhou, Xie et al. 2014). CD47, a well-known 'don't eat me' signal, controls erythrocyte lifespan positively through inhibition of phagocytosis via Signal regulatory protein (SIRPα)on normal/healthy erythrocytes, it was revealed an important rolein the clearance of agederythrocytes (Burger, de Korte et al. 2012). CD47 on erythrocytes and other cells can function as a regulator of target cell phagocytosis (Olsson, Nilsson et al. 2006). As a switch for erythrophagocytosis, CD47 undergoes a conformational change during ageing, which causes thrombospondin (TSP-1) binding and recognition of CD47 as an 'eat me' signal by SIRPα. The conformational status of CD47 can be changed through oxidative stress and binding of TSP-1 to apoptotic cells enhanced phagocytosis without inducing the secretion of pro-inflammatory cytokines (Burger, de Korte et al. 2012). CD47 expression was increased in the perihematomal white and gray matter after ICH, and deferoxamine treatment attenuated brain CD47 expression after ICH (Zhou, Xie et al. 2014). Higher microglial activation at day 3 after experimental ICH were foundafterCD47knockout blood injection, CD47has a key role in hematoma clearance after ICH (Ni, Mao et al. 2016). The present results of CD47 in ICH are confused and contradictory to its phagocytic property in pathological conditions, the exact role of CD47 in erythrocyte clearance after ICH still need to be further study.

3.3. Scavenger Receptor A (SRA)

Scavenger receptor A (SRA), also known as the macrophage scavenger receptor and cluster of differentiation 204 (CD204), a pattern recognition molecule, plays roles in lipid metabolism, atherogenesis, and a number of metabolic processes. SRA is a physiologic negative regulator of immune consequences. SRA is reported to be host protective in some disease states, but there is also compelling evidence that SRA plays a role in the pathophysiology of other diseases (Platt and Gordon 2001, Kelley, Ozment et al. 2014). On the one hand, SRA is clearly beneficial and/host protective in some models of disease. SRA on microglial cells mediates the binding of β amyloid fibrils and is responsible for preventing the accumulation of amyloid in the brain (El Khoury, Hickman et al. 1996). The decrease in SRA activity could contribute to the progression of neurodegeneration (Wilkinson and El Khoury 2012). SRA deficient mice exhibit impaired ability to control bacterial infections, resulting in increased mortality (Jozefowski 2012). SRA was highly expressed in erythrocyte lysate treated microglia. Genetic SRA ablation increased microglia activation and cytokine production, and sensitized mice to ICH induced neuron injury (Yang, Zhong et al. 2015). SRA down-regulated inflammatory response expression in microglia by suppressing TLR4-induced activation (Yuan, Shen et al. 2015). SRA could attenuate microglia mediated inflammation injury in ICH. In addition, SRA mediated negative feedback mechanism in neuroimmune homeostasis might provide a novel therapeutical strategy for ICH. Scavenger receptor SRA restrains T cell activation and protects against concanavalin A-induced hepatic injury (Yang, Zhong et al. 2015). SRA mediates activation of inflammatory signaling and apoptosis in ischemic stroke, both of which contribute to cerebral injury (Lu, Hua et al. 2010). The published data have given rise to an intriguing dilemma. As well as the other markers of Microglia/MMΦ activation, SRA is a two-edged sword in health and disease (Kelley, Ozment et al. 2014). Oxidized erythrocytes were internalized via SRA on macrophages, then sent to lysosomes for scavenging (Boyle, Johns et al. 2011). The exact role of SRA in ICH is dramatic and unclear, as a scavenger receptor it should participate in hematoma resolution through microglia activation and maybe produce undesirable inflammatory response, but the results of SRA in ICH is confusing (Yang, Zhong et al. 2015, Yuan, Shen et al. 2015).

3.4. Hp-Hb-CD163

After ICH, the cell-free Hb released from erythrocytes are first bound to haptoglobin (Hp), forming stable Hb-Hp complexes which are subsequently endocytosed by microglia/macrophages through the Hb scavenger receptor CD163. The clearance of Hb-Hp complexes from the hemolysis-affected environment is effectively mediated by circulating blood monocytes and tissue macrophages expressing CD163 (Zhao, Song et al. 2009).CD163 is a phagocytic marker and a hemoglobin scavenger receptor, of which expression is thought to be exclusive to perivascular (PVM) and monocyte- macrophage system (Graversen, Madsen et al. 2002, Fabriek, Van Haastert et al. 2005, Borda, Alvarez et al. 2008). It is a glycoprotein belonging to class B of the scavenger receptor cysteine rich superfamily. It functions as a membrane bound scavenger receptor for clearing extracellular haptoglobin-hemoglobin (Hp-Hb) complexes (Schaer, Alayash et al. 2007). As the most abundant erythrocyte protein, hemoglobin (Hb) is released into the extracellular space via complement-mediated cell lysis in the hours after ICH and is a potent mediator of oxidative stress induced blood-brain barrier disruption and brain injury (Hua, Xi et al. 2000, Wang, Mori et al. 2002, Katsu, Niizuma et al. 2010). Both in vitro and in vivo investigations have shown that ROS is highly produced after exposing Hb to cell culture or injecting Hb into mouse striatum (Wang, Mori et al. 2002, Qu, Chen et al. 2005). Haptoglobin (Hp) is the primary Hb-binding protein in human plasma, which attenuates the adverse biochemical and physiologic effects of extracellular Hb. The cellular receptor target of Hp is the monocyte/macrophage scavenger receptor, CD163 (Schaer, Vinchi et al. 2014). Excessive Hb upregulated expression of Hp and the Hb/Hp receptor CD163 in neurons in vivo and in vitro (Garton, He et al. 2016). A high expression of CD163 plays a major role in dampening the inflammatory response and in scavenging components of damaged cells. Free Hb binds to Hp and once Hp-Hb complex is endocytosed by CD163, which mediated delivery of Hb to the macrophage may fuel an anti-inflammatory response because heme metabolites have potent anti-inflammatory effects (Moestrup and Moller 2004).

3.5. Hx-Heme-LRP1

After ICH, the cell-free Hb and heme released from erythrocytes are first bound to haptoglobin (Hp) and hemopexin (Hx), forming stable Hb-Hp and heme-Hx complexes which are subsequently endocytosed by microglia/macrophages through the Hb scavenger receptor CD163 and the heme scavenger receptor CD91 respectively. With chronic hemolysis following ICH, Hp is depleted and Hb readily distributes to tissues where it might be exposed to oxidative conditions. In such conditions, heme can be released from ferric Hb. The free heme is highly toxic which can accelerate tissue damage by promoting peroxidative reactions and activation of inflammatory cascades (Ma, Day et al. 2016). The heme scavenger protein-hemopexin (Hx) contribute to hematoma removal as well as Hp-Hb after ICH (Aronowski and Zhao 2011), and Hx is another plasma glycoprotein able to bind heme with high affinity (Tolosano and Altruda 2002, Aronowski and Zhao 2011). Hx sequesters heme in an inert, non-toxic form and transports it to the liver for catabolism and excretion (Schaer, Vinchi et al. 2014). Hp and Hx have been characterized as a sequential defense system with Hp as the primary protector and Hx as a backup when Hp has been depleted during severe ICH. The linear relationship between Hx concentration and protection defined a highly efficient backup scavenger system during conditions of large excess of free Hb (Deuel, Vallelian et al. 2015). The heme-Hx complex is endocytosed by cells expressing the Low-density lipoprotein receptor-related protein-1 (LRP1) /CD91 receptor (Hvidberg, Maniecki et al. 2005, Wang, Manaenko et al. 2016). LRP1is a transmembrane receptor expressed on several cells types including macrophages, hepatocytes, neurons, vascular endothelial cells, pericytes, smooth muscle cells, and astrocytes (Zlokovic 2010, Sagare, Deane et al. 2012, Ramanathan, Nelson et al. 2015). Half of the BBB clearance is mediated by brain endothelial LRP1 in various model systems (Storck, Meister et al. 2016). As the only known endocytic receptor for Hx-heme complexes, LRP1 combined function of Hx may mediate localized heme clearance in the brain during cerebral hemorrhage (Hvidberg, Maniecki et al. 2005, Li, Saleem et al. 2009, Wang, Manaenko et al. 2016). Upon binding of heme-Hx to LRP-1, the complex becomes internalized via endocytosis into cells, inside the cell, the heme-Hx complex is dissociated by lysosomal activity. Heme is catabolized by heme oxygenases into biliverdin, carbon monoxide, and iron (Kumar and Bandyopadhyay 2005, Piccard, Van den Steen et al. 2007). Physiologic concentrations of hemopexin reduce peri-hematomal injury to an extent that is sufficient to ameliorate behavioral deficits in mice. These results suggest that hemopexin supplementation may be beneficial after hemorrhagic stroke (Chen, Zhang et al. 2011). There are indications that activation of LRP1 scavenging system in humans has favorable effects after subarachnoid hemorrhage (SAH) (Garland, Durnford et al. 2016). Recently we evaluated the effects of the activation of LRP1 system after ICH and confirmed that the activation of the LRP1 system is beneficial in experimental ICH (Wang, Manaenko et al. 2016). It should be proved in patients through above mentioned findings.

Taken together, the extravasated blood components (primarily erythrocytes lysis products) may be a major pathological factor after ICH, the activation of microglia/MMΦ phagocytic system through endogenous scavenger receptors maybe participate in hematoma/blood components resolution. Accordingly the activation of the scavenger receptors via pharmacological manipulations should be the future of targeted therapy in ICH.

4. The Upstream Regulatory Mechanism and Intervention Strategy for Scavenger Receptors after ICH

4.1. Nuclear Factor Erythroid 2-Related Factor 2 (Nrf2)

Nrf2 itself is a ubiquitous pleiotropic transcription factor and a pivotal mediator in redox homeostasis and inflammatory disorders, within the regulated region of many cytoprotective and antioxidant target genes which encode for critical mediators of cellular defense functions (Zhao, Hao et al. 2016). In unstressed conditions, Nrf2 is retained in the cytoplasm by its inhibitor kelch-like ECH-associated protein 1 (Keap1), upon activation by oxidative and electrophilic stress, Nrf2 disassociates from Keap1 and transactivates the antioxidant response element (ARE) then promotes the related cytoprotective pathways (Kensler, Wakabayashi et al. 2007). So Nrf2 is a key regulator of cellular resistance against oxidants (Ma 2013). In addition, the transcriptional activity of Nrf2 is essential for the clearance of phosphorylated tau via the selective autophagy (Jo, Gundemir et al. 2014). Also, knock-out of Nrf2 reduced the efficiency of macrophage accumulation and impaired clearance of myelin debris and phosphorylated tau (Zhang, Johnson et al. 2013, Kim, Choi et al. 2016). Nrf2, similar to transcription factor-peroxisome proliferator-activated receptor γ (PPAR-γ), controls the expression of CD36 (Ishii, Itoh et al. 2004, Maruyama, Tsukamoto et al. 2008), an essential scavenger receptor that in phagocytic cells assists in engulfment of various phagocytic targets (including extravascular/displaced RBC) which may represent a key component in attaining brain cleanup after stroke or intracerebral hemorrhage (Ren, Silverstein et al. 1995, Zhao, Grotta et al. 2009, Zhao, Sun et al. 2015). Removal of RBC by microglia and/or MMΦ may have a multiple indirect effect on oxidative stress, as it could reduce the accumulation of hemoglobin/heme/free iron (from lysed un-phagocytosed RBC) and consequently the formation of free radicals. Furthermore activated Nrf2 upregulated the levels of Hp in blood plasma and in ICH-affected brain in animals (Zhao and Aronowski 2013) as well as the expression of CD163 (Boyle, Johns et al. 2011).

In conclusion, Nrf2 in microglia/MMΦ plays a pivotal role in regulating the phagocytic functions of these cells and that in an experimental model of ICH, Nrf2 appears to be essential to hematoma clearance (Zhao, Sun et al. 2015). The potential role of Nrf2 following ICH were illustrated in Fig 9.

4.2. Peroxisome Proliferator-Activated Receptor -γ (PPAR-γ)

The peroxisome proliferator-activated receptor-gamma (PPAR-γ) is a ligand-activated transcription factor belonging to the nuclear hormone receptor superfamily and controlling reproduction, metabolism, development and immune response (Bernardo and Minghetti 2006). PPAR-γ expressed not only in adipocytes, but also in vascular tissues, such as vascular smooth muscle cells (VSMCs) and endothelial cells, and in macrophages (Ikeda, Sugawara et al. 2000). PPAR-γ and its agonists have a protective role in several neurological diseases via reducing inflammation (Abdelrahman, Sivarajah et al. 2005, Patzer, Zhao et al. 2008, Gamboa, Blankenship et al. 2010), decreasing oxidative damage (Zhao, Patzer et al. 2006, Gamboa, Blankenship et al. 2010), and attenuating cell death (Wu, Cheung et al. 2009). PPAR-γ is protective not only to neurons (Ou, Zhao et al. 2006, Zhao, Strong et al. 2009), astrocytes (Aleshin, Grabeklis et al. 2009, Wang, Zhao et al. 2010), oligodendrocytes (Hucke, Flossdorf et al. 2012), endothelia (Ramirez, Heilman et al. 2008), but also to microglia/ (**MMΦ**) (Petrova, Akama et al. 1999, Heneka, Sastre et al. 2005, Sauerbeck, Gao et al. 2011, Mandrekar-Colucci, Karlo et al. 2012) both in vitro and in vivo. PPAR-γ agonists reduce the ability of inflammatory stimuli to activate the alveolar macrophage while simultaneously stimulating phagocytosis of both opsonized and unopsonized particles, via the Fc-γ and CD36 receptors, respectively (Reddy 2008). PPAR-γ ligands have also been shown to upregulate the expression of scavenger receptor CD36 (Aronoff, Serezani et al. 2007)then promote microglia/macrophage-mediated clearance of toxic cellular debris (Moore, Rosen et al. 2001, Patel, Serghides et al. 2004, Majai, Sarang et al. 2007, Zhao, Sun et al. 2007). PPAR-γ induced CD36 expression may play an important role in stimulating phagocytotic efficacy of microglia (Zhao, Gonzales et al. 2015). PPAR-γ agonists not only increased microglia-mediated phagocytosis of RBC, but also reduced the production of H_2O_2 during the process of engulfment (Zhao, Sun et al. 2007, Zhao, Gonzales et al. 2015). As mentioned above the enhancement of phagocytosis by PPAR-γ agonists inevitably result in the inflammatory response and the dose-dependent neurotoxicity (Kondo, Shibata et al. 2002).

Some studies showed PPAR-γ had an interaction with Nrf2 (Ikeda, Sugawara et al. 2000, Satoh, Okamoto et al. 2006, Cho, Gladwell et al. 2010). Endogenous PPAR-γ ligands activities Nrf2 expression (Satoh, Okamoto et al. 2006), meanwhile Nrf2regulated PPAR-γ expression (Cho, Gladwell et al. 2010). Nrf2 controls CD36 expression independently of PPAR-γ (Olagnier, Lavergne et al. 2011). Expression of Nrf2 was reduced by knockdown of PPAR-γ, whereas PPAR-γ was reduced by knockdown of Nrf2, thereby demonstrating 2-way positive interactions. PPAR-γ agonists upregulate Nrf2 (Cho, Gladwell et al. 2010, Zhan, Zhang et al. 2012) and knockdown of PPAR-γ reduced the mRNA expression for Nrf2 (Luo, Aslam et al. 2015). This indicates a tight, positive, two-way reinforcing transcriptional interaction between PPAR-γ and Nrf2 that may improve endothelial function (Luo, Aslam et al. 2015). The interaction of PPAR-γ with Nrf2 following ICH were illustrated in Figure 9.

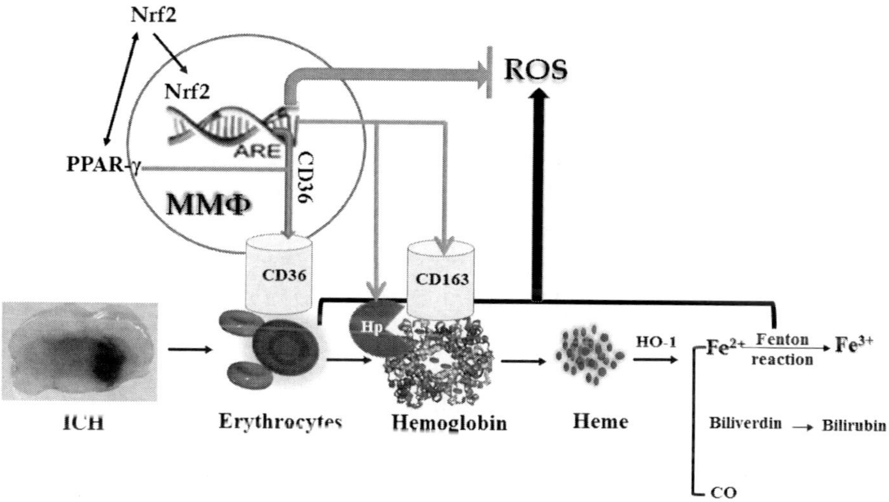

Figure 9. The potential function of the Nrf2/PPAR- γ pathway in brain following ICH.

5. Potential Exogenous Pharmacological/Molecular Manipulations Direct at Hematoma Resolution after ICH (as Illustrated in Figure 10)

5.1. Potential Treatment Options/Strategies for Hematoma Resolution via CD36

5.1.1. PPAR-γ Agonists

CD36 and catalase expression are regulated by PPAR-γ agonists (e.g., rosiglitazone). PPAR-γ agonist-induced upregulation of CD36 in macrophages enhances the ability of microglia to phagocytose red blood cells (in vitro assay), helps to improve hematoma resolution, and reduces ICH-induced deficit in a mouse model of ICH. In rat primary microglia in culture, PPAR-γ agonists not only increased microglia-mediated phagocytosis of RBC, but also reduced the production of H2O2 during the process of engulfment (Zhao, Sun et al. 2007). PPAR-γagonists could represent a potential treatment strategy for ICH (Zhao, Grotta et al. 2009).

Thiazolidinediones (e.g., ciglitazone, pioglitazone and rosiglitazone) are potent and selective activators of PPAR-γ (Lehmann, Moore et al. 1995). The derivatives of the parent compound thiazolidinedione such as rosiglitazone and pioglitazone are generally well-tolerated in AD and aMCI patients (Liu, Wang et al. 2015). The cyclopentanone prostaglandins (e.g., 15d–PGJ2) and monascinas well as thiazolidinediones are PPAR-γ agonists, which have been proven to act as potent and safe pro-survival factors for primary neurons subjected to either excitotoxic insult, oxygen-glucose deprivation (OGD) or H2O2-induced oxidative stress (Lehmann, Moore et al. 1995, Zhao, Zhang et al. 2006, Zhao, Gonzales et al. 2015) then attenuate ROS generation (Hsu, Lee et al. 2013). These PPAR-γ agonists are proposed to act as endogenous PPAR-γ ligands demonstrate rather limited selectivity toward PPAR-γ with some of its biological activation of Nrf2 (Satoh, Okamoto et al. 2006, Hsu, Lee et al. 2014). Monascin regulated PPAR-γ and Nrf-2 to improve lung oxidative inflammation (Hsu, Lee et al. 2014). Cilostazol, a potent phosphodiesterase type III inhibitor, has been used as a vasodilating antiplatelet drug for the treatment of ischemic symptoms in chronic peripheral arterial obstruction for preventing recurrence of cerebral infarction (Kambayashi, Liu et al. 2003). Cilostazol stimulates PPAR-γ transcriptional activity in human endothelial cells and may offer an effective therapeutic window along with complementary effects for individuals at high risk for type 2 diabetes by improving insulin sensitivity with anti-inflammatory effects (Park, Shin et al. 2009). Ankaflavin exerted PPAR-γ agonist activity by the upregulation of the signaling pathway of Nrf2 (Lee, Hsu et al. 2012).

The existing evidence showed that dose-dependent neurotoxicity of the 15d–PGJ2 in cerebellar granule cells, primary cortical neurons and spinal cord motor neurons (Rohn, Wong et al. 2001) which were believed to be associated with induction of apoptosis and not likely associated with the activation of PPAR-γ (Yagami, Ueda et al. 2003). On the other hand, the clinically relevant, more selective PPAR-γ agonist such as rosiglitazone, was linked to peripheral edema, increase in body weight, and cardiomyopathies and heart failure (Nissen and Wolski 2007). It is likely that PPAR-γ agonist treatment for ICH will be short-term, potentially avoiding these side effects, although this needs further testing.

5.1.2. Nrf2 Agonists

PPAR-γ controls expression of CD36 in macrophages, Nrf2 as a second important transcription factor involved in the induction of the scavenger receptor CD36 and antioxidant stress genes in atherosclerosis (Ishii, Itoh et al. 2004). Nrf2 transcription factor could be an alternative target to PPAR-γ in the control of severe malaria through parasite clearance (Olagnier, Lavergne et al. 2011). Nrf2 plays an essential role in the effective cleanup process after ICH, perhaps via coordinated efforts to enhance phagocytosis while concomitantly limiting oxidative stress (Zhao, Sun et al. 2015). Sulforaphane was capable of enhancing RBC phagocytosis and improving hematoma resolution via activating Nrf2 and inducing CD36 expression in microglias (Zhao, Sun et al. 2015). Monascin acts as a novel natural Nrf2 activator with PPAR-γ agonist activity were confirmed by Nrf2 and PPAR-γ reporter assays (Hsu, Lee et al. 2013). Protective effects of Ankaflavin against diabetes are mediated by the upregulation of the signaling pathway of Nrf2, which enhances antioxidant activity and serves as a PPAR-γ agonist to enhance insulin sensitivity (Lee, Hsu et al. 2012). Monascin and ankaflavin, the yellow pigments produced by Monascus species, have been proven to possess hypolipidemic functions and less side effects (Lee, Hung et al. 2013). Dimethyl fumarate is an orally administered fumarate ester recently FDA approved for first-line monotherapy of multiple sclerosis (Lundy, Wu et al. 2016), which stimulates Nrf2 activity to attenuate hyperphosphatamia in vitro or Vitamin D3-induced in vivo vascular calcification (Ha, Park et al. 2014). Carnosol increased the nuclear levels of Nrf2 (Martin, Rojo et al. 2004) and involved in the cytoprotective effects (Chen, Chen et al. 2011).

5.2. The Agonists for the Other Scavenger Receptors

5.2.1. CD163 Agonists

To date, the Hb-haptoglobin (Hp) complex is the only known ligand of CD163 (Kristiansen, Graversen et al. 2001, Madsen, Moller et al. 2004), and neither Hp alone nor free Hb has been found to display high-affinity binding to the receptor. Because the Hb-Hp complex binds to CD163 with high affinity and the receptor system has a high endocytotic capacity, CD163 is thought to mediate the clearance of Hb-Hp complexes from the blood (Moestrup and Moller 2004). Glucocorticoid can induce CD163 expression in macrophages enhances their capacity to bind and internalize Hb-Hp complexes (Schaer, Boretti et al. 2002).

5.2.2. Haptoglobin (Hp) and Hemopexin (Hx) Agonists

Nrf2 activator, Sulforaphane （SF）, used under conditions that reduced ICH-mediated brain damage is uniquely effective in mobilizing expression of Hp in the ICH-affected brain and peripheral blood. Similarly, SF applied to primary neuron-glial co-cultures under conditions demonstrated to increase Hp expression was effective in reducing damage to cultured cells subjected to ICH-like injury. These findings are overall consistent with the earlier studies identifying Hp as target of Nrf2, based on the transcriptional pattern of gene expression, in the small intestines of Nrf2 wild-type and -deficient mice (Zhao, Song et al. 2009). Hpexpressionis induced by inflammatory cytokines, dexamethasone and adrenoceptor agonists. In contrast, Hp was inhibited by nicotinic acid and the PPARγ agonist, rosiglitazone (do Nascimento, Hunter et al. 2004). The transcription rate of Hx increased by the calcium ionophore A23187, ionomycin, and phorbol 12-myristate 13-acetate (PMA) in serum-starved H4IIE rat hepatoma cells (Stred, Cote et al. 2003). Activated Nrf2 binds to antioxidant response elements (ARE), which promotes the transcription of haptoglobin and hemopexin (Belcher, Nath et al. 2013).

5.2.3. LRP1/CD91 Agonists

Low-density lipoprotein receptor-related protein-1(LRP1) contributed to heme clearance and blood-brain barrier protection after ICH in mice. The use of LRP1as supplement provides a novel approach to ameliorating intracerebral hemorrhage brain injury via its pleiotropic neuroprotective effects (Wang, Manaenko et al. 2016). Intrathecal infusions of CD91/LRP1 agonists- RBD (the Receptor Binding Domain of alpha-2-macroglobulin) or PEX (the hemopexin domain of MMP-9) in vitro significantly increases in axonal sprouting and regeneration after spinal cord injury via activating ERK and Akt pathway (Yoon, Van Niekerk et al. 2013). Imatinib promotes LRP1-dependent ERK activation and help to the pro-survival effects on β-cells (Fred, Boddeti et al. 2015). The upregulation of hepatic LRP1 also by rosiglitazone is mediated by PPAR-γ (Moon, Kim et al. 2012).

5.2.4. SR-A Agonists

Fucoidan, a SR-A agonist, could promote macrophage apoptosis by repressing ER stressor triggered autophagy (Huang, Li et al. 2014).Heptapeptide XD4 activates SR-A on the glia by increasing the binding of Aβ to SR-A, thereby promoting glial phagocytosis of Aβ oligomer in microglia and astrocytes (Zhang, Su et al. 2014).

5.2.5. CD47 Agonists

CD47 stimulated by its ligands-thrombospondins (TSPs), the agonist sequences occur in all five isoforms of TSP, it is possible that any TSP isoform could be proapoptotic (Manna and Frazier 2003). PKHB1, the serum-stable CD47 agonist peptide, might overcome drug refractoriness of chronic lymphocytic leukemia by the pro-apoptotic potential of targeting cell (Martinez-Torres, Quiney et al. 2015).

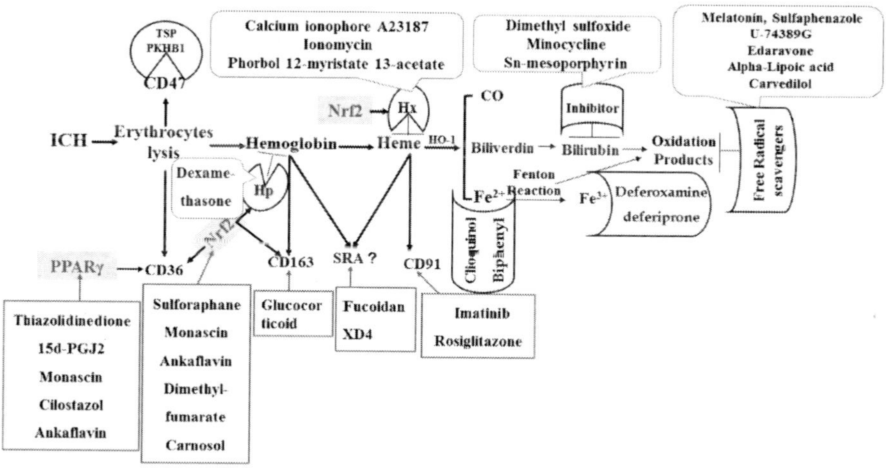

Figure 10. Intervention at facilitating hematoma resolution following ICH.

CONCLUSION

Taking together, most studies of hematoma clearance were in the clinical environment where intervention was surgery. However, there remain some indexes that should be considered for promoting hematoma resolution and removal. In this review, available information from understanding of the brain injury mechanisms underlying ICH to endogenous hematoma scavenging system are provided and potential intervention strategies discussed. Prospective study for hematoma resolution and how to speed up the process is more challengeable than reducing hematoma inflammation itself following acute ICH.

As a consequence of ICH, blood components enter brain parenchyma causing progressive damage to the surrounding brain. Unless hematoma is cleared, the reservoirs of blood continue to inflict injury to neurovascular structures and blunt the brain repair processes. So seeking and defining effective hematoma scavenger markers that can be intervened appropriately is meaningful for patients with ICH, which may contribute to improve outcomes in patients suffering from ICH.

REFERENCES

Abdelrahman, M., A. Sivarajah and C. Thiemermann (2005). "Beneficial effects of PPAR-gamma ligands in ischemia-reperfusion injury, inflammation and shock." *Cardiovasc Res* 65 (4): 772-781.

Albers, G. W. and P. Amarenco (2001). "Combination therapy with clopidogrel and aspirin: can the CURE results be extrapolated to cerebrovascula patients?" *Stroke* 32 (12): 2948-2949.

Albright, K. C., J. M. Burak, T. R. Chang, A. Aysenne, J. E. Siegler, L. Schluter, S. R. Martini, A. K. Boehme and S. Martin-Schild (2013). "*The Impact of Left Ventricular Hypertrophy and Diastolic Dysfunction on Outcome in Intracerebral Hemorrhage Patients.*" ISRN Stroke 2013.

Aleshin, S., S. Grabeklis, T. Hanck, M. Sergeeva and G. Reiser (2009). "Peroxisome proliferator-activated receptor (PPAR)-gamma positively controls and PPARalpha negatively controls cyclooxygenase-2 expression in rat brain astrocytes through a convergence on PPARbeta/delta via mutual control of PPAR expression levels." *Mol Pharmacol* 76 (2): 414-424.

Alexandrova, M. L. and M. P. Danovska (2011). "Serum C-reactive protein and lipid hydroperoxides in predicting short-term clinical outcome after spontaneous intracerebral hemorrhage." *J Clin Neurosci* 18 (2): 247-252.

Anderson, C. S., E. Heeley, Y. Huang, J. Wang, C. Stapf, C. Delcourt, R. Lindley, T. Robinson, P. Lavados, B. Neal, J. Hata, H. Arima, M. Parsons, Y. Li, J. Wang, S. Heritier, Q. Li, M. Woodward, R. J. Simes, S. M. Davis and J. Chalmers (2013). "Rapid blood-pressure lowering in patients with acute intracerebral hemorrhage." *N Engl J Med* 368 (25): 2355-2365.

Anderson, C. S., Y. Huang, J. G. Wang, H. Arima, B. Neal, B. Peng, E. Heeley, C. Skulina, M. W. Parsons, J. S. Kim, Q. L. Tao, Y. C. Li, J. D. Jiang, L. W. Tai, J. L. Zhang, E. Xu, Y. Cheng, S. Heritier, L. B. Morgenstern and J. Chalmers (2008). "Intensive blood pressure reduction in acute cerebral haemorrhage trial (INTERACT): a randomised pilot trial." *Lancet Neurol* 7 (5): 391-399.

Appelboom, G., M. Piazza, J. E. Han, S. S. Bruce, B. Hwang, A. Monahan, R. Y. Hwang, S. Kisslev, S. Mayer, P. M. Meyers, N. Badjatia and E. S. Connolly, Jr. (2013). "von Willebrand factor genetic variant associated with hematoma expansion after intracerebral hemorrhage." *J Stroke Cerebrovasc Dis* 22 (6): 713-717.

Aronoff, D. M., C. H. Serezani, J. K. Carstens, T. Marshall, S. R. Gangireddy, M. Peters-Golden and R. C. Reddy (2007). "Stimulatory Effects of Peroxisome Proliferator-Activated Receptor-gamma on Fcgamma Receptor-Mediated Phagocytosis by Alveolar Macrophages." *PPAR Res* 2007: 52546.

Aronowski, J. and C. E. Hall (2005). "New horizons for primary intracerebral hemorrhage treatment: experience from preclinical studies." *Neurol Res* 27 (3): 268-279.

Aronowski, J. and X. Zhao (2011). "Molecular pathophysiology of cerebral hemorrhage: secondary brain injury." *Stroke* 42 (6): 1781-1786.

Arslan, Y., T. K. Yoldas and Y. Zorlu (2013). "Interaction between vWF levels and aspirin resistance in ischemic stroke patients." *Transl Stroke Res* 4 (5): 484-487.

Asmis, L. M., I. Sulzer, M. Furlan and B. Lammle (2002). "Prekallikrein deficiency: the characteristic normalization of the severely prolonged aPTT following increased preincubation time is due to autoactivation of factor XII." *Thromb Res* 105 (6): 463-470.

Auer, L. M., W. Deinsberger, K. Niederkorn, G. Gell, R. Kleinert, G. Schneider, P. Holzer, G. Bone, M. Mokry, E. Korner and et al. (1989). "Endoscopic surgery versus medical treatment for spontaneous intracerebral hematoma: a randomized study." *J Neurosurg* 70 (4): 530-535.

Auriat, A. M., G. Silasi, Z. Wei, R. Paquette, P. Paterson, H. Nichol and F. Colbourne (2012). "Ferric iron chelation lowers brain iron levels after intracerebral hemorrhage in rats but does not improve outcome." Exp *Neurol* 234 (1): 136-143.

Aw, D. and J. C. Sharma (2012). "Antiplatelets in secondary stroke prevention: should clopidogrel be the first choice?" *Postgrad Med J* 88 (1035): 34-37.

Bagheri, M., J. R. Speakman, S. Shabbidar, F. Kazemi and K. Djafarian (2015). "A dose-response meta-analysis of the impact of body mass index on stroke and all-cause mortality in stroke patients: a paradox within a paradox." *Obes Rev* 16 (5): 416-423.

Baker, R. I., P. B. Coughlin, A. S. Gallus, P. L. Harper, H. H. Salem and E. M. Wood (2004). "Warfarin reversal: consensus guidelines, on behalf of the Australasian Society of Thrombosis and Haemostasis." *Med J Aust* 181 (9): 492-497.

Belcher, J. D., K. A. Nath and G. M. Vercellotti (2013). "Vasculotoxic and Proinflammatory Effects of Plasma Heme: Cell Signaling and Cytoprotective Responses." *ISRN Oxidative Med* 2013.

Bellander, B. M., S. K. Singhrao, M. Ohlsson, P. Mattsson and M. Svensson (2001). "Complement activation in the human brain after traumatic head injury." *J Neurotrauma* 18 (12): 1295-1311.

Bernardo, A. and L. Minghetti (2006). "PPAR-gamma agonists as regulators of microglial activation and brain inflammation." *Curr Pharm Des* 12 (1): 93-109.

Beshay, J. E., H. Morgan, C. Madden, W. Yu and R. Sarode (2010). "Emergency reversal of anticoagulation and antiplatelet therapies in neurosurgical patients." *J Neurosurg* 112 (2): 307-318.

Biffi, A., C. D. Anderson, J. M. Jagiella, H. Schmidt, B. Kissela, B. M. Hansen, J. Jimenez-Conde, C. R. Pires, A. M. Ayres, K. Schwab, L. Cortellini, J. Pera, A. Urbanik, J. M. Romero, N. S. Rost, J. N. Goldstein, A. Viswanathan, A. Pichler, C. Enzinger, R. Rabionet, B. Norrving, D. L. Tirschwell, M. Selim, D. L. Brown, S. L. Silliman, B. B. Worrall, J. F. Meschia, C. S. Kidwell, J. P. Broderick, S. M. Greenberg, J. Roquer, A. Lindgren, A. Slowik, R. Schmidt, D. Woo and J. Rosand (2011). "APOE genotype and extent of bleeding and outcome in lobar intracerebral haemorrhage: a genetic association study." *Lancet Neurol* 10 (8): 702-709.

Biffi, A., A. Sonni, C. D. Anderson, B. Kissela, J. M. Jagiella, H. Schmidt, J. Jimenez-Conde, B. M. Hansen, I. Fernandez-Cadenas, L. Cortellini, A. Ayres, K. Schwab, K. Juchniewicz, A. Urbanik, N. S. Rost, A. Viswanathan, T. Seifert-Held, E. M. Stoegerer, M. Tomas, R. Rabionet, X. Estivill, D. L. Brown, S. L. Silliman, M. Selim, B. B. Worrall, J. F. Meschia, J. Montaner, A. Lindgren, J. Roquer, R. Schmidt, S. M. Greenberg, A. Slowik, J. P. Broderick, D. Woo and J. Rosand (2010).

"Variants at APOE influence risk of deep and lobar intracerebral hemorrhage." *Ann Neurol* 68 (6): 934-943.

Bimpis, A., A. Papalois, K. Voumvourakis, O. Olah, L. Tiszlavicz and C. Liapi (2015). "Neuronal tumour necrosis factor-alpha and interleukin-1beta expression in a porcine model of intracerebral haemorrhage: Modulation by U-74389G." *Brain Res* 1615: 98-105.

Bjorkqvist, J., A. Jamsa and T. Renne (2013). "Plasma kallikrein: the bradykinin-producing enzyme." *Thromb Haemost* 110 (3): 399-407.

Borda, J. T., X. Alvarez, M. Mohan, A. Hasegawa, A. Bernardino, S. Jean, P. Aye and A. A. Lackner (2008). "CD163, a marker of perivascular macrophages, is up-regulated by microglia in simian immunodeficiency virus encephalitis after haptoglobin-hemoglobin complex stimulation and is suggestive of breakdown of the blood-brain barrier." *Am J Pathol* 172 (3): 725-737.

Boyle, J. J., M. Johns, J. Lo, A. Chiodini, N. Ambrose, P. C. Evans, J. C. Mason and D. O. Haskard (2011). "Heme induces heme oxygenase 1 via Nrf2: role in the homeostatic macrophage response to intraplaque hemorrhage." *Arterioscler Thromb Vasc Biol* 31 (11): 2685-2691.

Broderick, J., S. Connolly, E. Feldmann, D. Hanley, C. Kase, D. Krieger, M. Mayberg, L. Morgenstern, C. S. Ogilvy, P. Vespa and M. Zuccarello (2007). "Guidelines for the management of spontaneous intracerebral hemorrhage in adults: 2007 update: a guideline from the American Heart Association/American Stroke Association Stroke Council, High Blood Pressure Research Council, and the Quality of Care and Outcomes in Research Interdisciplinary Working Group." *Stroke* 38 (6): 2001-2023.

Broderick, J. P., M. N. Diringer, M. D. Hill, N. C. Brun, S. A. Mayer, T. Steiner, B. E. Skolnick and S. M. Davis (2007). "Determinants of intracerebral hemorrhage growth: an exploratory analysis." *Stroke* 38 (3): 1072-1075.

Brott, T., J. Broderick, R. Kothari, W. Barsan, T. Tomsick, L. Sauerbeck, J. Spilker, J. Duldner and J. Khoury (1997). "Early hemorrhage growth in patients with intracerebral hemorrhage." *Stroke* 28 (1): 1-5.

Brouwers, H. B., A. Biffi, A. M. Ayres, K. Schwab, L. Cortellini, J. M. Romero, N. S. Rost, A. Viswanathan, S. M. Greenberg, J. Rosand and J. N. Goldstein (2012). "Apolipoprotein E genotype predicts hematoma expansion in lobar intracerebral hemorrhage." *Stroke* 43 (6): 1490-1495.

Brouwers, H. B., J. N. Goldstein, J. M. Romero and J. Rosand (2012). "Clinical applications of the computed tomography angiography spot sign in acute intracerebral hemorrhage: a review." *Stroke* 43 (12): 3427-3432.

Brouwers, H. B. and S. M. Greenberg (2013). "Hematoma expansion following acute intracerebral hemorrhage." *Cerebrovasc Dis* 35 (3): 195-201.

Buehler, P. W., B. Abraham, F. Vallelian, C. Linnemayr, C. P. Pereira, J. F. Cipollo, Y. Jia, M. Mikolajczyk, F. S. Boretti, G. Schoedon, A. I. Alayash and D. J. Schaer (2009). "Haptoglobin preserves the CD163 hemoglobin scavenger pathway by shielding hemoglobin from peroxidative modification." *Blood* 113 (11): 2578-2586.

Burger, P., D. de Korte, T. K. van den Berg and R. van Bruggen (2012). "CD47 in Erythrocyte Ageing and Clearance – the Dutch Point of View." *Transfusion Medicine and Hemotherapy* 39 (5): 348-352.

Cairns, J. A., S. Connolly, S. McMurtry, M. Stephenson and M. Talajic (2011). "Canadian Cardiovascular Society atrial fibrillation guidelines 2010: prevention of stroke and systemic thromboembolism in atrial fibrillation and flutter." *Can J Cardiol* 27 (1): 74-90.

Caliaperumal, J., Y. Ma and F. Colbourne (2012). "Intra-parenchymal ferrous iron infusion causes neuronal atrophy, cell death and progressive tissue loss: implications for intracerebral hemorrhage." *Exp Neurol* 237 (2): 363-369.

Caliaperumal, J., S. Wowk, S. Jones, Y. Ma and F. Colbourne (2013). "Bipyridine, an iron chelator, does not lessen intracerebral iron-induced damage or improve outcome after intracerebral hemorrhagic stroke in rats." *Transl Stroke Res* 4 (6): 719-728.

Cao, D., J. Luo, D. Chen, H. Xu, H. Shi, X. Jing and W. Zang (2016). "CD36 regulates lipopolysaccharide-induced signaling pathways and mediates the internalization of Escherichia coli in cooperation with TLR4 in goat mammary gland epithelial cells." *Sci R*ep 6: 23132.

Chan, S. and J. C. Hemphill, 3rd (2014). "Critical care management of intracerebral hemorrhage." *Crit Care Clin* 30 (4): 699-717.

Chang, E. F., C. P. Claus, H. J. Vreman, R. J. Wong and L. J. Noble-Haeusslein (2005). "Heme regulation in traumatic brain injury: relevance to the adult and developing brain." *J Cereb Blood Flow Metab* 25 (11): 1401-1417.

Chen-Roetling, J., Y. Cai and R. F. Regan (2014). "Neuroprotective effect of heme oxygenase-2 knockout in the blood injection model of intracerebral hemorrhage." *BMC Res Notes* 7: 561.

Chen-Roetling, J., X. Lu and R. F. Regan (2015). "Targeting heme oxygenase after intracerebral hemorrhage." *Ther Targets Neurol* Dis 2 (1).

Chen, C. C., H. L. Chen, C. W. Hsieh, Y. L. Yang and B. S. Wung (2011). "Upregulation of NF-E2-related factor-2-dependent glutathione by carnosol provokes a cytoprotective response and enhances cell survival." *Acta Pharmacol Sin* 32 (1): 62-69.

Chen, L., X. Zhang, J. Chen-Roetling and R. F. Regan (2011). "Increased striatal injury and behavioral deficits after intracerebral hemorrhage in hemopexin knockout mice." *J Neurosurg* 114 (4): 1159-1167.

Chen, S., Q. Yang, G. Chen and J. H. Zhang (2015). "An update on inflammation in the acute phase of intracerebral hemorrhage." *Transl Stroke Res* 6 (1): 4-8.

Chen, S., L. Zeng and Z. Hu (2014). "Progressing haemorrhagic stroke: categories, causes, mechanisms and managements." *J Neurol* 261 (11): 2061-2078.

Chen, Y. C., C. M. Chen, J. L. Liu, S. T. Chen, M. L. Cheng and D. T. Chiu (2011). "Oxidative markers in spontaneous intracerebral hemorrhage: leukocyte 8-hydroxy-2'-deoxyguanosine as an independent predictor of the 30-day outcome." *J Neurosurg* 115 (6): 1184-1190.

Cheung, R. T. (1998). "Predictors of hematoma growth?" *Stroke* 29 (11): 2442-2443.

Cho, D. Y., C. C. Chen, W. Y. Lee, H. C. Lee and L. H. Ho (2008). "A new Modified Intracerebral Hemorrhage score for treatment decisions in basal ganglia hemorrhage--a randomized trial." *Crit Care Med* 36 (7): 2151-2156.

Cho, H. Y., W. Gladwell, X. Wang, B. Chorley, D. Bell, S. P. Reddy and S. R. Kleeberger (2010). "Nrf2-regulated PPAR{gamma} expression is critical to protection against acute lung injury in mice." *Am J Respir Crit Care Med* 182 (2): 170-182.

Chui, D. H., F. Marotta, M. L. Rao, D. S. Liu, S. C. Zhang and C. Ideo (1991). "Cholesterol-rich LDL perfused at physiological LDL-cholesterol concentration induces platelet aggregation and PAF-acetylhydrolase activation." *Biomed Pharmacother* 45 (1): 37-42.

Clark, J. F., M. Loftspring, W. L. Wurster, S. Beiler, C. Beiler, K. R. Wagner and G. J. Pyne-Geithman (2008). "Bilirubin oxidation products, oxidative stress, and intracerebral hemorrhage." *Acta Neurochir Suppl* 105: 7-12.

Clermont, A., T. J. Chilcote, T. Kita, J. Liu, P. Riva, S. Sinha and E. P. Feener (2011). "Plasma kallikrein mediates retinal vascular dysfunction and induces retinal thickening in diabetic rats." *Diabetes* 60 (5): 1590-1598.

Collis, R. E. and P. W. Collins (2015). "Haemostatic management of obstetric haemorrhage." *Anaesthesia* 70 Suppl 1: 78-86, e27-78.

D'Armiento, J., S. S. Dalal and K. Chada (1997). "Tissue, temporal and inducible expression pattern of haptoglobin in mice." *Gene* 195 (1): 19-27.

Danovska, M. (2010). "Alcohol Abuse Enhances Systemic Inflammatory Response in Patients after Spontaneous Intracerebral Haemorrhage." *Journal of IMAB - Annual Proceeding (Scientific Papers)* 16, book 3 (2010): 27-31.

Datla, S. R., G. J. Dusting, T. A. Mori, C. J. Taylor, K. D. Croft and F. Jiang (2007). "Induction of heme oxygenase-1 in vivo suppresses NADPH oxidase derived oxidative stress." *Hypertension* 50 (4): 636-642.

Davis, S. M., J. Broderick, M. Hennerici, N. C. Brun, M. N. Diringer, S. A. Mayer, K. Begtrup and T. Steiner (2006). "Hematoma growth is a determinant of mortality and poor outcome after intracerebral hemorrhage." *Neurology* 66 (8): 1175-1181.

De Lima, L. G., H. Saconato, A. N. Atallah and E. M. da Silva (2014). "Beta-blockers for preventing stroke recurrence." *Cochrane Database Syst Rev* (10): Cd007890.

Delcourt, C., Y. Huang, H. Arima, J. Chalmers, S. M. Davis, E. L. Heeley, J. Wang, M. W. Parsons, G. Liu and C. S. Anderson (2012). "Hematoma growth and outcomes in intracerebral hemorrhage: the INTERACT1 study." *Neurology* 79 (4): 314-319.

Delgado Almandoz, J. E., A. J. Yoo, M. J. Stone, P. W. Schaefer, A. Oleinik, H. B. Brouwers, J. N. Goldstein, J. Rosand, M. H. Lev, R. G. Gonzalez and J. M. Romero (2010). "The spot sign score in primary intracerebral hemorrhage identifies patients at highest risk of in-hospital mortality and poor outcome among survivors." *Stroke* 41 (1): 54-60.

Demchuk, A. M., D. Dowlatshahi, D. Rodriguez-Luna, C. A. Molina, Y. S. Blas, I. Dzialowski, A. Kobayashi, J. M. Boulanger, C. Lum, G. Gubitz, V. Padma, J. Roy, C. S. Kase, J. Kosior, R. Bhatia, S. Tymchuk, S. Subramaniam, D. J. Gladstone, M. D. Hill and R. I. Aviv (2012). "Prediction of haematoma growth and outcome in patients with intracerebral haemorrhage using the CT-angiography spot sign (PREDICT): a prospective observational study." *Lancet Neurol* 11 (4): 307-314.

Deuel, J. W., F. Vallelian, C. A. Schaer, M. Puglia, P. W. Buehler and D. J. Schaer (2015). "Different target specificities of haptoglobin and hemopexin define a sequential protection system against vascular hemoglobin toxicity." *Free Radic Biol Med* 89: 931-943.

Di Napoli, M., D. A. Godoy, V. Campi, M. del Valle, G. Pinero, M. Mirofsky, A. Popa-Wagner, L. Masotti, F. Papa and A. A. Rabinstein (2011). "C-reactive protein level measurement improves mortality prediction when added to the spontaneous intracerebral hemorrhage score." *Stroke* 42 (5): 1230-1236.

Di Napoli, M., D. A. Godoy, V. Campi, L. Masotti, C. J. Smith, A. R. Parry Jones, S. J. Hopkins, M. Slevin, F. Papa, L. Mogoanta, D. Pirici and A. Popa Wagner (2012). "C-reactive protein in intracerebral hemorrhage: time course, tissue localization, and prognosis." *Neurology* 79 (7): 690-699.

Di Napoli, M., A. R. Parry-Jones, C. J. Smith, S. J. Hopkins, M. Slevin, L. Masotti, V. Campi, P. Singh, F. Papa, A. Popa-Wagner, V. Tudorica and D. A. Godoy (2014). "C-reactive protein predicts hematoma growth in intracerebral hemorrhage." *Stroke* 45 (1): 59-65.

Ding, R., Y. Chen, S. Yang, X. Deng, Z. Fu, L. Feng, Y. Cai, M. Du, Y. Zhou and Y. Tang (2014). "Blood-brain barrier disruption induced by hemoglobin in vivo: Involvement of up-regulation of nitric oxide synthase and peroxynitrite formation." *Brain Res* 1571: 25-38.

Diringer, M. N. and D. F. Edwards (2001). "Admission to a neurologic/neurosurgical intensive care unit is associated with reduced mortality rate after intracerebral hemorrhage." *Crit Care Med* 29 (3): 635-640.

do Nascimento, C. O., L. Hunter and P. Trayhurn (2004). "Regulation of haptoglobin gene expression in 3T3-L1 adipocytes by cytokines, catecholamines, and PPARgamma." *Biochem Biophys Res Commun* 313 (3): 702-708.

Doens, D. and P. L. Fernandez (2014). "Microglia receptors and their implications in the response to amyloid beta for Alzheimer's disease pathogenesis." *J Neuroinflammation* 11: 48.

Du, Q., D. B. Yang, Y. F. Shen, W. H. Yu, Z. Y. Zhang, Q. Zhu, Z. H. Che, Q. J. Liu, H. Wang and X. Q. Dong (2013). "Plasma leptin level predicts hematoma growth and early neurological deterioration after acute intracerebral hemorrhage." *Peptides* 45: 35-39.

Ducruet, A. F., B. E. Zacharia, Z. L. Hickman, B. T. Grobelny, M. L. Yeh, S. A. Sosunov and E. S. Connolly, Jr. (2009). "The complement cascade as a therapeutic target in intracerebral hemorrhage." *Exp Neurol* 219 (2): 398-403.

El Khoury, J., S. E. Hickman, C. A. Thomas, L. Cao, S. C. Silverstein and J. D. Loike (1996). "Scavenger receptor-mediated adhesion of microglia to beta-amyloid fibrils." *Nature* 382 (6593): 716-719.

Emiru, T., E. M. Bershad, N. D. Zantek, Y. H. Datta, G. H. Rao, E. W. Hartley and A. A. Divani (2013). "Intracerebral hemorrhage: a review of coagulation function." *Clin Appl Thromb Hemost* 19 (6): 652-662.

Fabriek, B. O., E. S. Van Haastert, I. Galea, M. M. Polfliet, E. D. Dopp, M. M. Van Den Heuvel, T. K. Van Den Berg, C. J. De Groot, P. Van Der Valk and C. D. Dijkstra (2005). "CD163-positive perivascular macrophages in the human CNS express molecules for antigen recognition and presentation." *Glia* 51 (4): 297-305.

Fang, H., J. Chen, S. Lin, P. Wang, Y. Wang, X. Xiong and Q. Yang (2014). "CD36-mediated hematoma absorption following intracerebral hemorrhage: negative regulation by TLR4 signaling." *J Immunol* 192 (12): 5984-5992.

Fang, H., J. Chen, S. Lin, P. Wang, Y. Wang, X. Xiong and Q. Yang (2014). "CD36-Mediated Hematoma Absorption following Intracerebral Hemorrhage: Negative Regulation by TLR4 Signaling." *The Journal of Immunology Author Choice* 192 (12): 5984-5992.

Fang, H., P. F. Wang, Y. Zhou, Y. C. Wang and Q. W. Yang (2013). "Toll-like receptor 4 signaling in intracerebral hemorrhage-induced inflammation and injury." *J Neuroinflammation* 10: 27.

Feng, W., S. Tauhid, S. Goel, E. V. Sidorov and M. Selim (2012). "Hyperglycemia and outcome in intracerebral hemorrhage: from bedside to bench-more study is needed." *Transl Stroke Res* 3 (Suppl 1): 113-118.

Fred, R. G., S. K. Boddeti, M. Lundberg and N. Welsh (2015). "Imatinib mesylate stimulates low-density lipoprotein receptor-related protein 1-mediated ERK phosphorylation in insulin-producing cells." *Clin Sci (Lond)* 128 (1): 17-28.

Fuentes, B., M. A. Ortega-Casarrubios, P. Martinez and E. Diez-Tejedor (2007). "Action on vascular risk factors: importance of blood pressure and lipid lowering in stroke secondary prevention." *Cerebrovasc Dis* 24 Suppl 1: 96-106.

Fujii, Y., S. Takeuchi, O. Sasaki, T. Minakawa and R. Tanaka (1998). "Multivariate analysis of predictors of hematoma enlargement in spontaneous intracerebral hemorrhage." *Stroke* 29 (6): 1160-1166.

Gamboa, J., D. A. Blankenship, J. P. Niemi, G. E. Landreth, M. Karl, E. Hilow and S. Sundararajan (2010). "Extension of the neuroprotective time window for thiazolidinediones in ischemic stroke is dependent on time of reperfusion." *Neuroscience* 170 (3): 846-857.

Garland, P., A. J. Durnford, A. I. Okemefuna, J. Dunbar, J. A. Nicoll, J. Galea, D. Boche, D. O. Bulters and I. Galea (2016). "Heme-Hemopexin Scavenging Is Active in the Brain and Associates With Outcome After Subarachnoid Hemorrhage." *Stroke* 47 (3): 872-876.

Garton, T. P., Y. He, H. J. Garton, R. F. Keep, G. Xi and J. M. Strahle (2016). "Hemoglobin-induced neuronal degeneration in the hippocampus after neonatal intraventricular hemorrhage." *Brain Res* 1635: 86-94.

Geiger, A. S., A. C. Rice and S. M. Shapiro (2007). "Minocycline blocks acute bilirubin-induced neurological dysfunction in jaundiced Gunn rats." *Neonatology* 92 (4): 219-226.

Gioia, L. C., M. Kate, D. Dowlatshahi, M. D. Hill and K. Butcher (2015). "Blood pressure management in acute intracerebral hemorrhage: current evidence and ongoing controversies." *Curr Opin Crit Care* 21 (2): 99-106.

Goldstein, J. N., L. E. Fazen, R. Snider, K. Schwab, S. M. Greenberg, E. E. Smith, M. H. Lev and J. Rosand (2007). "Contrast extravasation on CT angiography predicts hematoma expansion in intracerebral hemorrhage." *Neurology* 68 (12): 889-894.

Gong, C., S. R. Ennis, J. T. Hoff and R. F. Keep (2001). "Inducible cyclooxygenase-2 expression after experimental intracerebral hemorrhage." *Brain Res* 901 (1-2): 38-46.

Gong, Y., G. Xi, H. Hu, Y. Gu, F. Huang, R. F. Keep and Y. Hua (2008). "Increase in brain thrombin activity after experimental intracerebral hemorrhage." *Acta Neurochir Suppl* 105: 47-50.

Gong, Y., G. H. Xi, R. F. Keep, J. T. Hoff and Y. Hua (2005). "Complement inhibition attenuates brain edema and neurological deficits induced by thrombin." *Acta Neurochir Suppl* 95: 389-392.

Gonzales, N. R., J. Shah, N. Sangha, L. Sosa, R. Martinez, L. Shen, M. Kasam, M. M. Morales, M. M. Hossain, A. D. Barreto, S. I. Savitz, G. Lopez, V. Misra, T. C. Wu, R. El Khoury, A. Sarraj, P. Sahota, W. Hicks, I. Acosta, M. R. Sline, M. H. Rahbar, X. Zhao, J. Aronowski and J. C. Grotta (2013). "Design of a prospective, dose-escalation study evaluating the Safety of Pioglitazone for Hematoma Resolution in Intracerebral Hemorrhage (SHRINC)." *Int J Stroke* 8 (5): 388-396.

Gonzalez-Moreno, E. I., C. R. Camara-Lemarroy, J. G. Gonzalez-Gonzalez and F. Gongora-Rivera (2014). "Glycemic variability and acute ischemic stroke: the missing link?" *Transl Stroke Res* 5 (6): 638-646.

Gordo, A. C., A. S. Falcao, A. Fernandes, M. A. Brito, R. F. Silva and D. Brites (2006). "Unconjugated bilirubin activates and damages microglia." *J Neurosci Res* 84 (1): 194-201.

Gravanis, I. and S. E. Tsirka (2005). "Tissue plasminogen activator and glial function." *Glia* 49 (2): 177-183.

Graversen, J. H., M. Madsen and S. K. Moestrup (2002). "CD163: a signal receptor scavenging haptoglobin-hemoglobin complexes from plasma." *Int J Biochem Cell Biol* 34 (4): 309-314.

Grivennikov, S. I. and M. Karin (2010). "Dangerous liaisons: STAT3 and NF-kappaB collaboration and crosstalk in cancer." *Cytokine Growth Factor Rev* 21 (1): 11-19.

Gu, S. J., H. F. Xuan, M. Lu, X. Z. Chen, W. F. Dong, X. F. Yan, Y. Si, G. L. Gao, D. X. Hu and J. Q. Miao (2013). "Admission plasma visfatin level strongly correlates with hematoma growth and early neurologic deterioration in patients with acute spontaneous basal ganglia hemorrhage." *Clin Chim Acta* 425: 85-89.

Gueders, M. M., J. M. Foidart, A. Noel and D. D. Cataldo (2006). "Matrix metalloproteinases (MMPs) and tissue inhibitors of MMPs in the respiratory tract: potential implications in asthma and other lung diseases." *Eur J Pharmacol* 533 (1-3): 133-144.

Guo, F., Y. Hua, J. Wang, R. F. Keep and G. Xi (2012). "Inhibition of carbonic anhydrase reduces brain injury after intracerebral hemorrhage." *Transl Stroke Res* 3 (1): 130-137.

Ha, C. M., S. Park, Y. K. Choi, J. Y. Jeong, C. J. Oh, K. H. Bae, S. J. Lee, J. H. Kim, K. G. Park, Y. Jun do and I. K. Lee (2014). "Activation of Nrf2 by dimethyl fumarate improves vascular calcification." *Vascul Pharmacol* 63 (1): 29-36.

Hama, S., Y. Ishihara, M. Watanabe, S. Danjo, Y. Nakamura and K. Itoh (2012). "Effects of sulfaphenazole after collagenase-induced experimental intracerebral hemorrhage in rats." *Biol Pharm Bull* 35 (10): 1849-1853.

Hanger, H. C., J. A. Geddes, T. J. Wilkinson, M. Lee and A. E. Baker (2013). "Warfarin-related intracerebral haemorrhage: better outcomes when reversal includes prothrombin complex concentrates." *Intern Med* J 43 (3): 308-316.

He, X. F., Y. Lan, Q. Zhang, D. X. Liu, Q. Wang, F. Y. Liang, J. S. Zeng, G. Q. Xu and Z. Pei (2016). "Deferoxamine inhibits microglial activation, attenuates blood-brain barrier disruption, rescues dendritic damage and improves spatial memory in a mouse model of microhemorrhages." *J Neurochem.*

Hemphill, J. C., 3rd, S. M. Greenberg, C. S. Anderson, K. Becker, B. R. Bendok, M. Cushman, G. L. Fung, J. N. Goldstein, R. L. Macdonald, P. H. Mitchell, P. A. Scott, M. H. Selim and D. Woo (2015). "Guidelines for the Management of Spontaneous Intracerebral Hemorrhage: A Guideline for Healthcare Professionals From the American Heart Association/American Stroke Association." *Stroke* 46 (7): 2032-2060.

Heneka, M. T., M. Sastre, L. Dumitrescu-Ozimek, A. Hanke, I. Dewachter, C. Kuiperi, K. O'Banion, T. Klockgether, F. Van Leuven and G. E. Landreth (2005). "Acute treatment with the PPARgamma agonist pioglitazone and ibuprofen reduces glial inflammation and Abeta1-42 levels in APPV717I transgenic mice." *Brain* 128 (Pt 6): 1442-1453.

Ho-Tin-Noe, B., M. Demers and D. D. Wagner (2011). "How platelets safeguard vascular integrity." *J Thromb Haemost* 9 Suppl 1: 56-65.

Hoj, L., V. Binder, F. Espersen, J. Greibe, S. N. Rasmussen and J. Rask-Madsen (1984). "Secretion rates of immunoglobulins, albumin, haptoglobin and complement factors C3 and C4 in the perfused jejunum and ileum of human Salmonella carriers." *Acta Pathol Microbiol Immunol Scand* C 92 (2): 129-132.

Hsu, J. C., C. Y. Hsieh, Y. H. Yang and C. Y. Lu (2015). "Net clinical benefit of oral anticoagulants: a multiple criteria decision analysis." *PLoS One 10* (4): e0124806.

Hsu, W. H., B. H. Lee, Y. Y. Chang, Y. W. Hsu and T. M. Pan (2013). "A novel natural Nrf2 activator with PPARgamma-agonist (monascin) attenuates the toxicity of methylglyoxal and hyperglycemia." *Toxicol Appl Pharmacol* 272 (3): 842-851.

Hsu, W. H., B. H. Lee, Y. W. Hsu and T. M. Pan (2013). "Peroxisome proliferator-activated receptor-gamma activators monascin and rosiglitazone attenuate carboxymethyllysine-induced fibrosis in hepatic stellate cells through regulating the oxidative stress pathway but independent of the receptor for advanced glycation end products signaling." *J Agric Food Chem* 61 (28): 6873-6879.

Hsu, W. H., B. H. Lee and T. M. Pan (2014). "Monascin attenuates oxidative stress-mediated lung inflammation via peroxisome proliferator-activated receptor-gamma (PPAR-gamma) and nuclear factor-erythroid 2 related factor 2 (Nrf-2) modulation." *J Agric Food Chem* 62 (23): 5337-5344.

Hu, X., P. Li, Y. Guo, H. Wang, R. K. Leak, S. Chen, Y. Gao and J. Chen (2012). "Microglia/macrophage polarization dynamics reveal novel mechanism of injury expansion after focal cerebral ischemia." *Stroke* 43 (11): 3063-3070.

Hu, X., C. Tao, Q. Gan, J. Zheng, H. Li and C. You (2016). "Oxidative Stress in Intracerebral Hemorrhage: Sources, Mechanisms, and Therapeutic Targets." *Oxidative Medicine and Cellular Longevity* 2016: 3215391.

Hu, X., C. Tao, Q. Gan, J. Zheng, H. Li and C. You (2016). "Oxidative Stress in Intracerebral Hemorrhage: Sources, Mechanisms, and Therapeutic Targets." *Oxid Med Cell Longev* 2016: 3215391.

Hua, Y., R. F. Keep, J. T. Hoff and G. Xi (2007). "Brain injury after intracerebral hemorrhage: the role of thrombin and iron." *Stroke* 38 (2 Suppl): 759-762.

Hua, Y., G. Xi, R. F. Keep and J. T. Hoff (2000). "Complement activation in the brain after experimental intracerebral hemorrhage." *J Neurosurg* 92 (6): 1016-1022.

Huang, F. P., G. Xi, R. F. Keep, Y. Hua, A. Nemoianu and J. T. Hoff (2002). "Brain edema after experimental intracerebral hemorrhage: role of hemoglobin degradation products." *J Neurosurg* 96 (2): 287-293.

Huang, H., X. Li, Y. Zhuang, N. Li, X. Zhu, J. Hu, J. Ben, Q. Yang, H. Bai and Q. Chen (2014). "Class A scavenger receptor activation inhibits endoplasmic reticulum stress-induced autophagy in macrophage." *J Biomed Res* 28 (3): 213-221.

Huang, Q., W. M. Dai, Y. Q. Jie, G. F. Yu, X. F. Fan and A. Wu (2013). "High concentrations of visfatin in the peripheral blood of patients with acute basal ganglia hemorrhage are associated with poor outcome." *Peptides* 39: 55-58.

Hucke, S., J. Flossdorf, B. Grutzke, I. R. Dunay, K. Frenzel, J. Jungverdorben, B. Linnartz, M. Mack, M. Peitz, O. Brustle, C. Kurts, T. Klockgether, H. Neumann, M. Prinz, H. Wiendl, P. Knolle and L. Klotz (2012). "Licensing of myeloid cells promotes central nervous system autoimmunity and is controlled by peroxisome proliferator-activated receptor gamma." *Brain 135* (Pt 5): 1586-1605.

Hunter, C. A. and S. A. Jones (2015). "IL-6 as a keystone cytokine in health and disease." *Nat Immunol* 16 (5): 448-457.

Husemann, J., J. D. Loike, R. Anankov, M. Febbraio and S. C. Silverstein (2002). "Scavenger receptors in neurobiology and neuropathology: their role on microglia and other cells of the nervous system." *Glia* 40 (2): 195-205.

Huttner, H. B., P. D. Schellinger, M. Hartmann, M. Kohrmann, E. Juettler, J. Wikner, S. Mueller, U. Meyding-Lamade, R. Strobl, U. Mansmann, S. Schwab and T. Steiner (2006). "Hematoma growth and outcome in treated neurocritical care patients with intracerebral hemorrhage related to oral anticoagulant therapy: comparison of acute treatment strategies using vitamin K, fresh frozen plasma, and prothrombin complex concentrates." *Stroke* 37 (6): 1465-1470.

Hvidberg, V., M. B. Maniecki, C. Jacobsen, P. Hojrup, H. J. Moller and S. K. Moestrup (2005). "Identification of the receptor scavenging hemopexin-heme complexes." *Blood* 106 (7): 2572-2579.

Ikeda, Y., A. Sugawara, Y. Taniyama, A. Uruno, K. Igarashi, S. Arima, S. Ito and K. Takeuchi (2000). "Suppression of rat thromboxane synthase gene transcription by peroxisome proliferator-activated receptor gamma in macrophages via an interaction with NRF2." *J Biol Chem* 275 (42): 33142-33150.

Ishii, T., K. Itoh, E. Ruiz, D. S. Leake, H. Unoki, M. Yamamoto and G. E. Mann (2004). "Role of Nrf2 in the regulation of CD36 and stress protein expression in murine macrophages: activation by oxidatively modified LDL and 4-hydroxynonenal." *Circ Res* 94 (5): 609-616.

Iso, H., S. Sato, A. Kitamura, Y. Naito, T. Shimamoto and Y. Komachi (2003). "Fat and protein intakes and risk of intraparenchymal hemorrhage among middle-aged Japanese." *Am J Epidemiol* 157 (1): 32-39.

James, R. F., V. Palys, J. R. Lomboy, J. R. Lamm, Jr. and S. D. Simon (2013). "The role of anticoagulants, antiplatelet agents, and their reversal strategies in the management of intracerebral hemorrhage." *Neurosurg Focus* 34 (5): E6.

Jauch, E. C., C. J. Lindsell, O. Adeoye, J. Khoury, W. Barsan, J. Broderick, A. Pancioli and T. Brott (2006). "Lack of evidence for an association between hemodynamic variables and hematoma growth in spontaneous intracerebral hemorrhage." *Stroke* 37 (8): 2061-2065.

Jo, C., S. Gundemir, S. Pritchard, Y. N. Jin, I. Rahman and G. V. Johnson (2014). "Nrf2 reduces levels of phosphorylated tau protein by inducing autophagy adaptor protein NDP52." *Nat Commun* 5: 3496.

Jozefowski, S. (2012). "[The role of the class A scavenger receptors, SR-A and MARCO, in the immune system. Part 2. Contribution to recognition and phagocytosis of pathogens as well as induction of immune response]." *Postepy Hig Med Dosw* (Online) 66: 120-131.

Jung, K. H., K. Chu, S. T. Lee, S. J. Kim, E. C. Song, E. H. Kim, D. K. Park, D. I. Sinn, J. M. Kim, M. Kim and J. K. Roh (2007). "Blockade of AT1 receptor reduces apoptosis, inflammation, and oxidative stress in normotensive rats with intracerebral hemorrhage." *J Pharmacol Exp Ther* 322 (3): 1051-1058.

Kambayashi, J., Y. Liu, B. Sun, Y. Shakur, M. Yoshitake and F. Czerwiec (2003). "Cilostazol as a unique antithrombotic agent." *Curr Pharm* Des 9 (28): 2289-2302.

Katsu, M., K. Niizuma, H. Yoshioka, N. Okami, H. Sakata and P. H. Chan (2010). "Hemoglobin-induced oxidative stress contributes to matrix metalloproteinase activation and blood-brain barrier dysfunction in vivo." *J Cereb Blood Flow Metab* 30 (12): 1939-1950.

Katsuki, H. (2010). "Exploring neuroprotective drug therapies for intracerebral hemorrhage." *J Pharmacol Sci* 114 (4): 366-378.

Kawanishi, M., N. Kawai, T. Nakamura, C. Luo, T. Tamiya and S. Nagao (2008). "Effect of delayed mild brain hypothermia on edema formation after intracerebral hemorrhage in rats." *J Stroke Cerebrovasc Dis* 17 (4): 187-195.

Kazui, S., K. Minematsu, H. Yamamoto, T. Sawada and T. Yamaguchi (1997). "Predisposing factors to enlargement of spontaneous intracerebral hematoma." *Stroke* 28 (12): 2370-2375.

Keep, R. F., Y. Hua and G. Xi (2012). "Intracerebral haemorrhage: mechanisms of injury and therapeutic targets." *Lancet Neurol* 11 (8): 720-731.

Kelley, J. L., T. R. Ozment, C. Li, J. B. Schweitzer and D. L. Williams (2014). "Scavenger Receptor-A (CD204): A Two-Edged Sword in Health and Disease." *Critical reviews in immunology* 34 (3): 241-261.

Kelley, J. L., T. R. Ozment, C. Li, J. B. Schweitzer and D. L. Williams (2014). "Scavenger receptor-A (CD204): a two-edged sword in health and disease." *Crit Rev Immunol* 34 (3): 241-261.

Kensler, T. W., N. Wakabayashi and S. Biswal (2007). "Cell survival responses to environmental stresses via the Keap1-Nrf2-ARE pathway." *Annu Rev Pharmacol Toxicol* 47: 89-116.

Kernan, W. N., B. Ovbiagele, H. R. Black, D. M. Bravata, M. I. Chimowitz, M. D. Ezekowitz, M. C. Fang, M. Fisher, K. L. Furie, D. V. Heck, S. C. Johnston, S. E. Kasner, S. J. Kittner, P. H. Mitchell, M. W. Rich, D. Richardson, L. H. Schwamm and J. A. Wilson (2014). "Guidelines for the prevention of stroke in patients with stroke and transient ischemic attack: a guideline for healthcare professionals from the American Heart Association/American Stroke Association." *Stroke* 45 (7): 2160-2236.

Keynes, R. G. and J. Garthwaite (2004). "Nitric oxide and its role in ischaemic brain injury." *Curr Mol Med* 4 (2): 179-191.

Kim, C. K., W. S. Ryu, I. Y. Choi, Y. J. Kim, D. Rim, B. J. Kim, H. Jang, B. W. Yoon and S. H. Lee (2013). "Detrimental effects of leptin on intracerebral hemorrhage via the STAT3 signal pathway." *J Cereb Blood Flow Metab* 33 (6): 944-953.

Kim, S., K. J. Choi, S. J. Cho, S. M. Yun, J. P. Jeon, Y. H. Koh, J. Song, G. V. Johnson and C. Jo (2016). "Fisetin stimulates autophagic degradation of phosphorylated tau via the activation of TFEB and Nrf2 transcription factors." *Sci Rep* 6: 24933.

Koch, S., J. G. Romano, A. M. Forteza, C. M. Otero and A. A. Rabinstein (2008). "Rapid blood pressure reduction in acute intracerebral hemorrhage: feasibility and safety." *Neurocrit Care* 8 (3): 316-321.

Kondo, M., T. Shibata, T. Kumagai, T. Osawa, N. Shibata, M. Kobayashi, S. Sasaki, M. Iwata, N. Noguchi and K. Uchida (2002). "15-Deoxy-Delta (12,14)-prostaglandin J (2): the endogenous electrophile that induces neuronal apoptosis." *Proc Natl Acad Sci USA* 99 (11): 7367-7372.

Kristiansen, M., J. H. Graversen, C. Jacobsen, O. Sonne, H. J. Hoffman, S. K. Law and S. K. Moestrup (2001). "Identification of the haemoglobin scavenger receptor." *Nature* 409 (6817): 198-201.

Kumar, S. and U. Bandyopadhyay (2005). "Free heme toxicity and its detoxification systems in human." *Toxicol Lett* 157 (3): 175-188.

Kuramatsu, J. B., S. T. Gerner, P. D. Schellinger, J. Glahn, M. Endres, J. Sobesky, J. Flechsenhar, H. Neugebauer, E. Juttler, A. Grau, F. Palm, J. Rother, P. Michels, G. F. Hamann, J. Huwel, G. Hagemann, B. Barber, C. Terborg, F. Trostdorf, H. Bazner, A. Roth, J. Wohrle, M. Keller, M. Schwarz, G. Reimann, J. Volkmann, W. Mullges, P. Kraft, J. Classen, C. Hobohm, M. Horn, A. Milewski, H. Reichmann, H. Schneider, E. Schimmel, G. R. Fink, C. Dohmen, H. Stetefeld, O. Witte, A. Gunther, T. Neumann-Haefelin, A. E. Racs, M. Nueckel, F. Erbguth, S. P. Kloska, A. Dorfler, M. Kohrmann, S. Schwab and H. B. Huttner (2015). "Anticoagulant reversal, blood pressure levels, and anticoagulant resumption in patients with anticoagulation-related intracerebral hemorrhage." *Jama* 313 (8): 824-836.

Kuramatsu, J. B., H. B. Huttner and S. Schwab (2013). "Advances in the management of intracerebral hemorrhage." *J Neural Transm* (Vienna) 120 Suppl 1: S35-41.

Kwon, K. J., J. N. Kim, M. K. Kim, S. Y. Kim, K. S. Cho, S. J. Jeon, H. Y. Kim, J. H. Ryu, S. Y. Han, J. H. Cheong, L. J. Ignarro, S. H. Han and C. Y. Shin (2013). "Neuroprotective effects of valproic acid against hemin toxicity: possible involvement of the down-regulation of heme oxygenase-1 by regulating ubiquitin-proteasomal pathway." *Neurochem Int* 62 (3): 240-250.

Kwon, K. J., J. N. Kim, M. K. Kim, J. Lee, L. J. Ignarro, H. J. Kim, C. Y. Shin and S. H. Han (2011). "Melatonin synergistically increases resveratrol-induced heme oxygenase-1 expression through the inhibition of ubiquitin-dependent proteasome pathway: a possible role in neuroprotection." *J Pineal Res* 50 (2): 110-123.

Lagasse, H. A., I. U. Anidi, J. M. Craig, N. Limjunyawong, A. K. Poupore, W. Mitzner and A. L. Scott (2015). "Recruited monocytes modulate malaria-induced lung injury through CD36-mediated clearance of sequestered infected erythrocytes." *J Leukoc Biol.*

Lakovic, K., J. Ai, J. D'Abbondanza, A. Tariq, M. Sabri, A. K. Alarfaj, P. Vasdev and R. L. Macdonald (2014). "Bilirubin and its oxidation products damage brain white matter." *J Cereb Blood Flow Metab* 34 (11): 1837-1847.

Le Roux, P., C. V. Pollack, Jr., M. Milan and A. Schaefer (2014). "Race against the clock: overcoming challenges in the management of anticoagulant-associated intracerebral hemorrhage." *J Neurosurg* 121 Suppl: 1-20.

Lee, B. H., W. H. Hsu, Y. Y. Chang, H. F. Kuo, Y. W. Hsu and T. M. Pan (2012). "Ankaflavin: a natural novel PPARgamma agonist upregulates Nrf2 to attenuate methylglyoxal-induced diabetes in vivo." *Free Radic Biol Med* 53 (11): 2008-2016.

Lee, C. L., Y. P. Hung, Y. W. Hsu and T. M. Pan (2013). "Monascin and ankaflavin have more anti-atherosclerosis effect and less side effect involving increasing creatinine phosphokinase activity than monacolin K under the same dosages." *J Agric Food Chem* 61 (1): 143-150.

Lee, S. T., K. Chu, K. H. Jung, J. Kim, E. H. Kim, S. J. Kim, D. I. Sinn, S. Y. Ko, M. Kim and J. K. Roh (2006). "Memantine reduces hematoma expansion in experimental intracerebral hemorrhage, resulting in functional improvement." *J Cereb Blood Flow Metab* 26 (4): 536-544.

Lehmann, J. M., L. B. Moore, T. A. Smith-Oliver, W. O. Wilkison, T. M. Willson and S. A. Kliewer (1995). "An antidiabetic thiazolidinedione is a high affinity ligand for peroxisome proliferator-activated receptor gamma (PPAR gamma)." *J Biol Chem* 270 (22): 12953-12956.

Lei, B., B. Mace, S. T. Bellows, P. M. Sullivan, M. P. Vitek, D. T. Laskowitz and M. L. James (2012). "Interaction between sex and apolipoprotein e genetic background in a murine model of intracerebral hemorrhage." *Transl Stroke Res* 3 (1): 94-101.

Lekic, T., R. Hartman, H. Rojas, A. Manaenko, W. Chen, R. Ayer, J. Tang and J. H. Zhang (2010). "Protective effect of melatonin upon neuropathology, striatal function, and memory ability after intracerebral hemorrhage in rats." *J Neurotrauma* 27 (3): 627-637.

Levy, J. H. and L. T. Goodnough (2015). "How I use fibrinogen replacement therapy in acquired bleeding." *Blood* 125 (9): 1387-1393.

Li, Q., Y. J. Huang, G. Zhang, F. J. Lv, X. Wei, M. X. Dong, J. J. Chen, L. J. Zhang, X. Y. Qin and P. Xie (2015). "Intraventricular Hemorrhage and Early Hematoma Expansion in Patients with Intracerebral Hemorrhage." *Sci Rep* 5: 11357.

Li, R. C., S. Saleem, G. Zhen, W. Cao, H. Zhuang, J. Lee, A. Smith, F. Altruda, E. Tolosano and S. Dore (2009). "Heme-hemopexin complex attenuates neuronal cell death and stroke damage." *J Cereb Blood Flow Metab* 29 (5): 953-964.

Li, T. T., M. L. Fan, S. X. Hou, X. Y. Li, D. M. Barry, H. Jin, S. Y. Luo, F. Kong, L. F. Lau, X. R. Dai, G. H. Zhang and L. L. Zhou (2015). "A novel snake venom-derived GPIb antagonist, anfibatide, protects mice from acute experimental ischaemic stroke and reperfusion injury." *Br J Pharmacol* 172 (15): 3904-3916.

Liew, H. K., C. Y. Pang, C. W. Hsu, M. J. Wang, T. Y. Li, H. F. Peng, J. S. Kuo and J. Y. Wang (2012). "Systemic administration of urocortin after intracerebral hemorrhage reduces neurological deficits and neuroinflammation in rats." *J Neuroinflammation* 9: 13.

Lim, J. K., H. S. Hwang, B. M. Cho, H. K. Lee, S. K. Ahn, S. M. Oh and S. K. Choi (2008). "Multivariate analysis of risk factors of hematoma expansion in spontaneous intracerebral hemorrhage." *Surg Neurol* 69 (1): 40-45; discussion 45.

Lin, S., Q. Yin, Q. Zhong, F. L. Lv, Y. Zhou, J. Q. Li, J. Z. Wang, B. Y. Su and Q. W. Yang (2012). "Heme activates TLR4-mediated inflammatory injury via MyD88/TRIF signaling pathway in intracerebral hemorrhage." *J Neuroinflammation* 9: 46.

Lipton, S. A. (2007). "Pathologically-activated therapeutics for neuroprotection: mechanism of NMDA receptor block by memantine and S-nitrosylation." *Curr Drug Targets* 8 (5): 621-632.

Liu, C. M., B. Z. Shi and J. S. Zhou (2014). "Effects of thrombin on the secondary cerebral injury of perihematomal tissues of rats after intracerebral hemorrhage." *Genet Mol Res* 13 (2): 4617-4626.

Liu, D., T. Cheng, H. Guo, J. A. Fernandez, J. H. Griffin, X. Song and B. V. Zlokovic (2004). "Tissue plasminogen activator neurovascular toxicity is controlled by activated protein C." *Nat Med* 10 (12): 1379-1383.

Liu, J., B. B. Gao, A. C. Clermont, P. Blair, T. J. Chilcote, S. Sinha, R. Flaumenhaft and E. P. Feener (2011). "Hyperglycemia-induced cerebral hematoma expansion is mediated by plasma kallikrein." *Nat Med* 17 (2): 206-210.

Liu, J., B. B. Gao and E. P. Feener (2010). "Proteomic identification of novel plasma kallikrein substrates in the astrocyte secretome." *Transl Stroke Res* 1 (4): 276-286.

Liu, J., L. N. Wang and J. P. Jia (2015). "Peroxisome proliferator-activated receptor-gamma agonists for Alzheimer's disease and amnestic mild cognitive impairment: a systematic review and meta-analysis." *Drugs Aging* 32 (1): 57-65.

Liu, X. C., L. Y. Jing, M. F. Yang, K. Wang, Y. Wang, X. Y. Fu, J. Fang, Y. J. Hou, J. Y. Sun, D. W. Li, Z. Y. Zhang, L. L. Mao, Y. M. Tang, X. T. Fu, C. D. Fan, X. Y. Yang and B. L. Sun (2016). "Enhanced Neuroprotection of Minimally Invasive Surgery Joint Local Cooling Lavage against ICH-induced Inflammation Injury and Apoptosis in Rats." *Cell Mol Neurobiol* 36 (5): 647-655.

Loftspring, M. C., H. L. Johnson, R. Feng, A. J. Johnson and J. F. Clark (2011). "Unconjugated bilirubin contributes to early inflammation and edema after intracerebral hemorrhage." *J Cereb Blood Flow Metab* 31 (4): 1133-1142.

Lu, C., F. Hua, L. Liu, T. Ha, J. Kalbfleisch, J. Schweitzer, J. Kelley, R. Kao, D. Williams and C. Li (2010). "Scavenger receptor class-A has a central role in cerebral ischemia-reperfusion injury." *J Cereb Blood Flow Metab* 30 (12): 1972-1981.

Lukic-Panin, V., K. Deguchi, T. Yamashita, J. Shang, X. Zhang, F. Tian, N. Liu, H. Kawai, T. Matsuura and K. Abe (2010). "Free radical scavenger edaravone administration protects against tissue plasminogen activator induced oxidative stress and blood brain barrier damage." *Curr Neurovasc Res* 7 (4): 319-329.

Lundy, S. K., Q. Wu, Q. Wang, C. A. Dowling, S. H. Taitano, G. Mao and Y. Mao-Draayer (2016). "Dimethyl fumarate treatment of relapsing-remitting multiple sclerosis influences B-cell subsets." *Neurol Neuroimmunol Neuroinflamm* 3 (2): e211.

Luo, Z., S. Aslam, W. J. Welch and C. S. Wilcox (2015). "Activation of nuclear factor erythroid 2-related factor 2 coordinates dimethylarginine dimethylaminohydrolase/PPAR-gamma/endothelial nitric oxide synthase pathways that enhance nitric oxide generation in human glomerular endothelial cells." *Hypertension* 65 (4): 896-902.

Ma, B., J. P. Day, H. Phillips, B. Slootsky, E. Tolosano and S. Dore (2016). "Deletion of the hemopexin or heme oxygenase-2 gene aggravates brain injury following stroma-free hemoglobin-induced intracerebral hemorrhage." *J Neuroinflammation* 13 (1): 26.

Ma, Q. (2013). "Role of nrf2 in oxidative stress and toxicity." *Annu Rev Pharmacol Toxicol* 53: 401-426.

Madsen, M., H. J. Moller, M. J. Nielsen, C. Jacobsen, J. H. Graversen, T. van den Berg and S. K. Moestrup (2004). "Molecular characterization of the haptoglobin. hemoglobin receptor CD163. Ligand binding properties of the scavenger receptor cysteine-rich domain region." *J Biol Chem* 279 (49): 51561-51567.

Majai, G., Z. Sarang, K. Csomos, G. Zahuczky and L. Fesus (2007). "PPARgamma-dependent regulation of human macrophages in phagocytosis of apoptotic cells." *Eur J Immunol* 37 (5): 1343-1354.

Makogonenko, E., G. Tsurupa, K. Ingham and L. Medved (2002). "Interaction of fibrin (ogen) with fibronectin: further characterization and localization of the fibronectin-binding site." *Biochemistry* 41 (25): 7907-7913.

Mandrekar-Colucci, S., J. C. Karlo and G. E. Landreth (2012). "Mechanisms underlying the rapid peroxisome proliferator-activated receptor-gamma-mediated amyloid clearance and reversal of cognitive deficits in a murine model of Alzheimer's disease." *J Neurosci* 32 (30): 10117-10128.

Manna, P. P. and W. A. Frazier (2003). "The mechanism of CD47-dependent killing of T cells: heterotrimeric Gi-dependent inhibition of protein kinase A." *J Immunol* 170 (7): 3544-3553.

Mannucci, P. M., Z. M. Ruggeri, F. I. Pareti and A. Capitanio (1977). "1-Deamino-8-d-arginine vasopressin: a new pharmacological approach to the management of haemophilia and von Willebrands' diseases." *Lancet* 1 (8017): 869-872.

Mannucci, P. M. and A. Tripodi (2012). "Hemostatic defects in liver and renal dysfunction." Hematology Am Soc Hematol Educ Program 2012: 168-173.

Manzanero, S., T. Santro and T. V. Arumugam (2013). "Neuronal oxidative stress in acute ischemic stroke: sources and contribution to cell injury." *Neurochem Int* 62 (5): 712-718.

Marti-Fabregas, J., M. Borrell, Y. Silva, R. Delgado-Mederos, S. Martinez-Ramirez, M. de Juan-Delago, I. Tirado, A. Alejaldre, R. Marin, J. L. Marti-Vilalta and J. Fontcuberta (2010). "Hemostatic proteins and their association with hematoma growth in patients with acute intracerebral hemorrhage." *Stroke* 41 (12): 2976-2978.

Martin, D., A. I. Rojo, M. Salinas, R. Diaz, G. Gallardo, J. Alam, C. M. De Galarreta and A. Cuadrado (2004). "Regulation of heme oxygenase-1 expression through the phosphatidylinositol 3-kinase/Akt pathway and the Nrf2 transcription factor in response to the antioxidant phytochemical carnosol." *J Biol Chem* 279 (10): 8919-8929.

Martinez-Torres, A. C., C. Quiney, T. Attout, H. Boullet, L. Herbi, L. Vela, S. Barbier, D. Chateau, E. Chapiro, F. Nguyen-Khac, F. Davi, M. Le Garff-Tavernier, R. Moumne, M. Sarfati, P. Karoyan, H. Merle-Beral, P. Launay and S. A. Susin (2015). "CD47 agonist peptides induce programmed cell death in refractory chronic lymphocytic leukemia B cells via PLCgamma1 activation: evidence from mice and humans." *PLoS Med* 12 (3): e1001796.

Maruyama, A., S. Tsukamoto, K. Nishikawa, A. Yoshida, N. Harada, K. Motojima, T. Ishii, A. Nakane, M. Yamamoto and K. Itoh (2008). "Nrf2 regulates the alternative first exons of CD36 in macrophages through specific antioxidant response elements." *Arch Biochem Biophys* 477 (1): 139-145.

Mates, J. M., J. A. Segura, F. J. Alonso and J. Marquez (2012). "Oxidative stress in apoptosis and cancer: an update." *Arch Toxicol* 86 (11): 1649-1665.

Mayer, S. A., N. C. Brun, K. Begtrup, J. Broderick, S. Davis, M. N. Diringer, B. E. Skolnick and T. Steiner (2008). "Efficacy and safety of recombinant activated factor VII for acute intracerebral hemorrhage." *N Engl J Med* 358 (20): 2127-2137.

Mendelow, A. D., B. A. Gregson, E. N. Rowan, G. D. Murray, A. Gholkar and P. M. Mitchell (2013). "Early surgery versus initial conservative treatment in patients with spontaneous supratentorial lobar intracerebral haematomas (STICH II): a randomised trial." *Lancet* 382 (9890): 397-408.

Mendelow, A. D. and A. Unterberg (2007). "Surgical treatment of intracerebral haemorrhage." *Curr Opin Crit Care* 13 (2): 169-174.

Meretoja, A., L. Churilov, B. C. Campbell, R. I. Aviv, N. Yassi, C. Barras, P. Mitchell, B. Yan, H. Nandurkar, C. Bladin, T. Wijeratne, N. J. Spratt, J. Jannes, J. Sturm, J. Rupasinghe, J. Zavala, A. Lee, T. Kleinig, R. Markus, C. Delcourt, N. Mahant, M. W. Parsons, C. Levi, C. S. Anderson, G. A. Donnan and S. M. Davis (2014). "The spot sign and tranexamic acid on preventing ICH growth--AUStralasia Trial (STOP-AUST): protocol of a phase II randomized, placebo-controlled, double-blind, multicenter trial." *Int J Stroke* 9 (4): 519-524.

Mingam, R., A. Moranis, R. M. Bluthe, V. De Smedt-Peyrusse, K. W. Kelley, P. Guesnet, M. Lavialle, R. Dantzer and S. Laye (2008). "Uncoupling of interleukin-6 from its signalling pathway by dietary n-3-polyunsaturated fatty acid deprivation alters sickness behaviour in mice." *Eur J Neurosci* 28 (9): 1877-1886.

Moestrup, S. K. and H. J. Moller (2004). "CD163: a regulated hemoglobin scavenger receptor with a role in the anti-inflammatory response." *Ann Med* 36 (5): 347-354.

Montanola, A., S. F. de Retana, A. Lopez-Rueda, C. Merino-Zamorano, A. Penalba, P. Fernandez-Alvarez, D. Rodriguez-Luna, A. Malagelada, F. Pujadas, J. Montaner and M. Hernandez-Guillamon (2016). "ApoA1, ApoJ and ApoE Plasma Levels and Genotype Frequencies in Cerebral Amyloid Angiopathy." *Neuromolecular Med* 18 (1): 99-108.

Moon, J. H., H. J. Kim, H. M. Kim, A. H. Yang, B. W. Lee, E. S. Kang, H. C. Lee and B. S. Cha (2012). "Upregulation of hepatic LRP1 by rosiglitazone: a possible novel mechanism of the beneficial effect of thiazolidinediones on atherogenic dyslipidemia." *J Mol Endocrinol* 49 (3): 165-174.

Moore, K. J., E. D. Rosen, M. L. Fitzgerald, F. Randow, L. P. Andersson, D. Altshuler, D. S. Milstone, R. M. Mortensen, B. M. Spiegelman and M. W. Freeman (2001). "The role of PPAR-gamma in macrophage differentiation and cholesterol uptake." *Nat Med* 7 (1): 41-47.

Morawo, A. O. and E. J. Gilmore (2016). "Critical Care Management of Intracerebral Hemorrhage." *Semin Neurol* 36 (3): 225-232.

Morgenstern, L. B., A. M. Demchuk, D. H. Kim, R. F. Frankowski and J. C. Grotta (2001). "Rebleeding leads to poor outcome in ultra-early craniotomy for intracerebral hemorrhage." *Neurology* 56 (10): 1294-1299.

Morgenstern, L. B., R. F. Frankowski, P. Shedden, W. Pasteur and J. C. Grotta (1998). "Surgical treatment for intracerebral hemorrhage (STICH): a single-center, randomized clinical trial." *Neurology* 51 (5): 1359-1363.

Morotti, A., M. J. Jessel, H. B. Brouwers, G. J. Falcone, K. Schwab, A. M. Ayres, A. Vashkevich, C. D. Anderson, A. Viswanathan, S. M. Greenberg, M. E. Gurol, J. M. Romero, J. Rosand and J. N. Goldstein (2016). "CT Angiography Spot Sign, Hematoma Expansion, and Outcome in Primary Pontine Intracerebral Hemorrhage." *Neurocrit Care*.

Mracsko, E., E. Javidi, S. Y. Na, A. Kahn, A. Liesz and R. Veltkamp (2014). "Leukocyte invasion of the brain after experimental intracerebral hemorrhage in mice." *Stroke* 45 (7): 2107-2114.

Mracsko, E. and R. Veltkamp (2014). "Neuroinflammation after intracerebral hemorrhage." *Front Cell Neurosci* 8: 388.

Munoz-Sanchez, J. and M. E. Chanez-Cardenas (2014). "A review on hemeoxygenase-2: focus on cellular protection and oxygen response." *Oxid Med Cell Longev* 2014: 604981.

Naidech, A. M., B. Jovanovic, S. Liebling, R. K. Garg, S. L. Bassin, B. R. Bendok, R. A. Bernstein, M. J. Alberts and H. H. Batjer (2009). "Reduced platelet activity is associated with early clot growth and worse 3-month outcome after intracerebral hemorrhage." *Stroke* 40 (7): 2398-2401.

Naidech, A. M., M. B. Maas, K. E. Levasseur-Franklin, E. M. Liotta, J. C. Guth, M. Berman, J. M. Rosenow, P. F. Lindholm, B. R. Bendok, S. Prabhakaran, R. A. Bernstein and H. C. Kwaan (2014). "Desmopressin improves platelet activity in acute intracerebral hemorrhage." *Stroke* 45 (8): 2451-2453.

Nakamura, T., R. F. Keep, Y. Hua, J. T. Hoff and G. Xi (2005). "Oxidative DNA injury after experimental intracerebral hemorrhage." *Brain Res* 1039 (1-2): 30-36.

Nakamura, T., R. F. Keep, Y. Hua, S. Nagao, J. T. Hoff and G. Xi (2006). "Iron-induced oxidative brain injury after experimental intracerebral hemorrhage." *Acta Neurochir Suppl* 96: 194-198.

Nakamura, T., G. Xi, Y. Hua, T. Schallert, J. T. Hoff and R. F. Keep (2004). "Intracerebral hemorrhage in mice: model characterization and application for genetically modified mice." *J Cereb Blood Flow Metab* 24 (5): 487-494.

Nandi, D., P. Tahiliani, A. Kumar and D. Chandu (2006). "The ubiquitin-proteasome system." J Biosci 31 (1): 137-155.

Newell, D. W., M. M. Shah, R. Wilcox, D. R. Hansmann, E. Melnychuk, J. Muschelli and D. F. Hanley (2011). "Minimally invasive evacuation of spontaneous intracerebral hemorrhage using sonothrombolysis." *J Neurosurg* 115 (3): 592-601.

Ni, W., S. Mao, G. Xi, R. F. Keep and Y. Hua (2016). "Role of Erythrocyte CD47 in Intracerebral Hematoma Clearance." *Stroke* 47 (2): 505-511.

Nicole, O., F. Docagne, C. Ali, I. Margaill, P. Carmeliet, E. T. MacKenzie, D. Vivien and A. Buisson (2001). "The proteolytic activity of tissue-plasminogen activator enhances NMDA receptor-mediated signaling." *Nat Med* 7 (1): 59-64.

NINDS ICH Workshop Participants (2005). "Priorities for clinical research in intracerebral hemorrhage: report from a National Institute of Neurological Disorders and Stroke workshop." *Stroke* 36 (3): e23-41.

Nissen, S. E. and K. Wolski (2007). "Effect of rosiglitazone on the risk of myocardial infarction and death from cardiovascular causes." *N Engl J Med* 356 (24): 2457-2471.

Noda, H., H. Iso, F. Irie, T. Sairenchi, E. Ohtaka, M. Doi, Y. Izumi and H. Ohta (2009). "Low-density lipoprotein cholesterol concentrations and death due to intraparenchymal hemorrhage: the Ibaraki Prefectural Health Study." *Circulation* 119 (16): 2136-2145.

O'Shaughnessy, D. F., C. Atterbury, P. Bolton Maggs, M. Murphy, D. Thomas, S. Yates and L. M. Williamson (2004). "Guidelines for the use of fresh-frozen plasma, cryoprecipitate and cryosupernatant." *Br J Haematol* 126 (1): 11-28.

Ohwaki, K., E. Yano, H. Nagashima, M. Hirata, T. Nakagomi and A. Tamura (2004). "Blood pressure management in acute intracerebral hemorrhage: relationship between elevated blood pressure and hematoma enlargement." *Stroke* 35 (6): 1364-1367.

Olagnier, D., R. A. Lavergne, E. Meunier, L. Lefevre, C. Dardenne, A. Aubouy, F. Benoit-Vical, B. Ryffel, A. Coste, A. Berry and B. Pipy (2011). "Nrf2, a PPARgamma alternative pathway to promote CD36 expression on inflammatory macrophages: implication for malaria." *PLoS Pathog* 7 (9): e1002254.

Olsson, M., A. Nilsson and P. A. Oldenborg (2006). "Target cell CD47 regulates macrophage activation and erythrophagocytosis." *Transfus Clin Biol* 13 (1-2): 39-43.

Ooneda, G., Y. Yoshida, K. Suzuki, H. Shinkai, S. Hori, K. Kobori, Y. Takayama and M. Sekiguchi (1978). "Smooth muscle cells in the development of plasmatic arterionecrosis, arteriosclerosis, and arterial contraction." *Blood Vessels* 15 (1-3): 148-156.

Osuka, K., Y. Watanabe, N. Usuda, K. Atsuzawa, H. Shima, M. Takeuchi, M. Yasuda and M. Takayasu (2013). "Activation of JAK-STAT3 signaling pathway in chronic subdural hematoma outer membranes." *Neurosci Lett* 534: 166-170.

Ou, Z., X. Zhao, L. A. Labiche, R. Strong, J. C. Grotta, O. Herrmann and J. Aronowski (2006). "Neuronal expression of peroxisome proliferator-activated receptor-gamma (PPARgamma) and 15d-prostaglandin J2--mediated protection of brain after experimental cerebral ischemia in rat." *Brain Res* 1096 (1): 196-203.

Ovesen, C., I. Havsteen, S. Rosenbaum and H. Christensen (2014). "Prediction and observation of post-admission hematoma expansion in patients with intracerebral hemorrhage." *Front Neurol* 5: 186.

Pabinger, I., B. Brenner, U. Kalina, S. Knaub, A. Nagy and H. Ostermann (2008). "Prothrombin complex concentrate (Beriplex P/N) for emergency anticoagulation reversal: a prospective multinational clinical trial." *J Thromb Haemost* 6 (4): 622-631.

Pandey, A. S. and G. Xi (2014). "Intracerebral hemorrhage: a multimodality approach to improving outcome." *Transl Stroke Res* 5 (3): 313-315.

Park, S. Y., H. K. Shin, J. H. Lee, C. D. Kim, W. S. Lee, B. Y. Rhim and K. W. Hong (2009). "Cilostazol ameliorates metabolic abnormalities with suppression of proinflammatory markers in a db/db mouse model of type 2 diabetes via activation of peroxisome proliferator-activated receptor gamma transcription." *J Pharmacol Exp Ther* 329 (2): 571-579.

Patel, S. N., L. Serghides, T. G. Smith, M. Febbraio, R. L. Silverstein, T. W. Kurtz, M. Pravenec and K. C. Kain (2004). "CD36 mediates the phagocytosis of Plasmodium falciparum-infected erythrocytes by rodent macrophages." *J Infect Dis* 189 (2): 204-213.

Patzer, A., Y. Zhao, I. Stock, P. Gohlke, T. Herdegen and J. Culman (2008). "Peroxisome proliferator-activated receptorsgamma (PPARgamma) differently modulate the interleukin-6 expression in the peri-infarct cortical tissue in the acute and delayed phases of cerebral ischaemia." *Eur J Neurosci* 28 (9): 1786-1794.

Peeling, J., H. J. Yan, S. G. Chen, M. Campbell and M. R. Del Bigio (1998). "Protective effects of free radical inhibitors in intracerebral hemorrhage in rat." *Brain Res* 795 (1-2): 63-70.

Petrova, T. V., K. T. Akama and L. J. Van Eldik (1999). "Cyclopentenone prostaglandins suppress activation of microglia: down-regulation of inducible nitric-oxide synthase by 15-deoxy-Delta12,14-prostaglandin J2." *Proc Natl Acad Sci USA* 96 (8): 4668-4673.

Petzold, A., G. Keir, M. Kerr, A. Kay, N. Kitchen, M. Smith and E. J. Thompson (2006). "Early identification of secondary brain damage in subarachnoid hemorrhage: a role for glial fibrillary acidic protein." *J Neurotrauma* 23 (7): 1179-1184.

Phipps, J. A., A. C. Clermont, S. Sinha, T. J. Chilcote, S. E. Bursell and E. P. Feener (2009). "Plasma kallikrein mediates angiotensin II type 1 receptor-stimulated retinal vascular permeability." *Hypertension* 53 (2): 175-181.

Piccard, H., P. E. Van den Steen and G. Opdenakker (2007). "Hemopexin domains as multifunctional liganding modules in matrix metalloproteinases and other proteins." *J Leukoc Biol* 81 (4): 870-892.

Platt, N. and S. Gordon (2001). "Is the class A macrophage scavenger receptor (SR-A) multifunctional? - The mouse's tale." *J Clin Invest* 108 (5): 649-654.

Prasad, K., A. D. Mendelow and B. Gregson (2008). "Surgery for primary supratentorial intracerebral haemorrhage." *Cochrane Database Syst Rev* (4): Cd000200.

Priglinger, M., H. Arima, C. Anderson and M. Krause (2015). "No relationship of lipid-lowering agents to hematoma growth: pooled analysis of the intensive blood pressure reduction in acute cerebral hemorrhage trials studies." *Stroke* 46 (3): 857-859.

Przybylowski, C. J., D. Ding, R. M. Starke, R. Webster Crowley and K. C. Liu (2015). "Endoport-assisted surgery for the management of spontaneous intracerebral hemorrhage." *J Clin Neurosci* 22 (11): 1727-1732.

Qing, W. G., Y. Q. Dong, T. Q. Ping, L. G. Lai, L. D. Fang, H. W. Min, L. Xia and P. Y. Heng (2009). "Brain edema after intracerebral hemorrhage in rats: the role of iron overload and aquaporin 4." *J Neurosurg* 110 (3): 462-468.

Qu, Y., J. Chen, L. Benvenisti-Zarom, X. Ma and R. F. Regan (2005). "Effect of targeted deletion of the heme oxygenase-2 gene on hemoglobin toxicity in the striatum." *J Cereb Blood Flow Metab* 25 (11): 1466-1475.

Qureshi, A. I., A. D. Mendelow and D. F. Hanley (2009). "Intracerebral haemorrhage." *Lancet* 373 (9675): 1632-1644.

Qureshi, A. I., Y. Y. Palesch, R. Martin, J. Novitzke, S. Cruz-Flores, A. Ehtisham, M. A. Ezzeddine, J. N. Goldstein, J. F. Kirmani, H. M. Hussein, M. F. Suri, N. Tariq and Y. Liu (2011). "Association of serum glucose concentrations during acute hospitalization with hematoma expansion, perihematomal edema, and three month outcome among patients with intracerebral hemorrhage." *Neurocrit Care* 15 (3): 428-435.

Radmanesh, F., G. J. Falcone, C. D. Anderson, T. W. Battey, A. M. Ayres, A. Vashkevich, K. A. McNamara, K. Schwab, J. M. Romero, A. Viswanathan, S. M. Greenberg, J. N. Goldstein, J. Rosand and H. B. Brouwers (2014). "Risk factors for computed tomography angiography spot sign in deep and lobar intracerebral hemorrhage are shared." *Stroke* 45 (6): 1833-1835.

Rahpeymai, Y., M. A. Hietala, U. Wilhelmsson, A. Fotheringham, I. Davies, A. K. Nilsson, J. Zwirner, R. A. Wetsel, C. Gerard, M. Pekny and M. Pekna (2006). "Complement: a novel factor in basal and ischemia-induced neurogenesis." *Embo j* 25 (6): 1364-1374.

Ramanathan, A., A. R. Nelson, A. P. Sagare and B. V. Zlokovic (2015). "Impaired vascular-mediated clearance of brain amyloid beta in Alzheimer's disease: the role, regulation and restoration of LRP1." *Front Aging Neurosci 7*: 136.

Ramirez, S. H., D. Heilman, B. Morsey, R. Potula, J. Haorah and Y. Persidsky (2008). "Activation of peroxisome proliferator-activated receptor gamma (PPARgamma) suppresses Rho GTPases in human brain microvascular endothelial cells and inhibits adhesion and transendothelial migration of HIV-1 infected monocytes." *J Immunol* 180 (3): 1854-1865.

Rannikmae, K., R. N. Kalaria, S. M. Greenberg, H. C. Chui, F. A. Schmitt, N. Samarasekera, R. Al-Shahi Salman and C. L. Sudlow (2014). "APOE associations with severe CAA-associated vasculopathic changes: collaborative meta-analysis." *J Neurol Neurosurg Psychiatry* 85 (3): 300-305.

Rashid, P., J. Leonardi-Bee and P. Bath (2003). "Blood pressure reduction and secondary prevention of stroke and other vascular events: a systematic review." *Stroke* 34 (11): 2741-2748.

Reddy, R. C. (2008). "Immunomodulatory role of PPAR-gamma in alveolar macrophages." J Investig Med 56 (2): 522-527.

Ren, Y., R. L. Silverstein, J. Allen and J. Savill (1995). "CD36 gene transfer confers capacity for phagocytosis of cells undergoing apoptosis." *J Exp Med* 181 (5): 1857-1862.

Ribo, M. and J. C. Grotta (2006). “Latest advances in intracerebral hemorrhage.” *Curr Neurol Neurosci Rep* 6 (1): 17-22.

Rincon, F. and S. A. Mayer (2008). “Clinical review: Critical care management of spontaneous intracerebral hemorrhage.” *Crit Care* 12 (6): 237.

Rincon, F. and S. A. Mayer (2012). “Intracerebral hemorrhage: clinical overview and pathophysiologic concepts.” *Transl Stroke Res* 3 (Suppl 1): 10-24.

Rodriguez-Luna, D., S. Pineiro, M. Rubiera, M. Ribo, P. Coscojuela, J. Pagola, A. Flores, M. Muchada, B. Ibarra, P. Meler, E. Sanjuan, M. Hernandez-Guillamon, J. Alvarez-Sabin, J. Montaner and C. A. Molina (2013). “Impact of blood pressure changes and course on hematoma growth in acute intracerebral hemorrhage.” *Eur J Neurol* 20 (9): 1277-1283.

Rodriguez-Luna, D., M. Rubiera, M. Ribo, P. Coscojuela, J. Pagola, S. Pineiro, B. Ibarra, P. Meler, O. Maisterra, F. Romero, J. Alvarez-Sabin and C. A. Molina (2011). “Serum low-density lipoprotein cholesterol level predicts hematoma growth and clinical outcome after acute intracerebral hemorrhage.” *Stroke* 42 (9): 2447-2452.

Rohn, T. T., S. M. Wong, C. W. Cotman and D. H. Cribbs (2001). “15-deoxy-delta12,14-prostaglandin J2, a specific ligand for peroxisome proliferator-activated receptor-gamma, induces neuronal apoptosis.” *Neuroreport* 12 (4): 839-843.

Rolland, W. B., T. Lekic, P. R. Krafft, Y. Hasegawa, O. Altay, R. Hartman, R. Ostrowski, A. Manaenko, J. Tang and J. H. Zhang (2013). “Fingolimod reduces cerebral lymphocyte infiltration in experimental models of rodent intracerebral hemorrhage.” *Exp Neurol* 241: 45-55.

Ruff, C. T., R. P. Giugliano, E. Braunwald, D. A. Morrow, S. A. Murphy, J. F. Kuder, N. Deenadayalu, P. Jarolim, J. Betcher, M. Shi, K. Brown, I. Patel, M. Mercuri and E. M. Antman (2015). “Association between edoxaban dose, concentration, anti-Factor Xa activity, and outcomes: an analysis of data from the randomised, double-blind ENGAGE AF-TIMI 48 trial.” *Lancet* 385 (9984): 2288-2295.

Rynkowski, M. A., G. H. Kim, M. C. Garrett, B. E. Zacharia, M. L. Otten, S. A. Sosunov, R. J. Komotar, B. G. Hassid, A. F. Ducruet, J. D. Lambris and E. S. Connolly (2009). “C3a receptor antagonist attenuates brain injury after intracerebral hemorrhage.” *J Cereb Blood Flow Metab* 29 (1): 98-107.

Rynkowski, M. A., G. H. Kim, R. J. Komotar, M. L. Otten, A. F. Ducruet, B. E. Zacharia, C. P. Kellner, D. K. Hahn, M. B. Merkow, M. C. Garrett, R. M. Starke, B. M. Cho, S. A. Sosunov and E. S. Connolly (2008). "A mouse model of intracerebral hemorrhage using autologous blood infusion." *Nat Protoc* 3 (1): 122-128.

Sadler, J. E. (1998). "Biochemistry and genetics of von Willebrand factor." *Annu Rev Biochem* 67: 395-424.

Sagare, A. P., R. Deane and B. V. Zlokovic (2012). "Low-density lipoprotein receptor-related protein 1: a physiological Abeta homeostatic mechanism with multiple therapeutic opportunities." *Pharmacol Ther* 136 (1): 94-105.

Sahni, R. and J. Weinberger (2007). "Management of intracerebral hemorrhage." *Vasc Health Risk Manag* 3 (5): 701-709.

Sansing, L. H., T. H. Harris, F. A. Welsh, S. E. Kasner, C. A. Hunter and K. Kariko (2011). "Toll-like receptor 4 contributes to poor outcome after intracerebral hemorrhage." *Ann Neurol* 70 (4): 646-656.

Satoh, T., S. I. Okamoto, J. Cui, Y. Watanabe, K. Furuta, M. Suzuki, K. Tohyama and S. A. Lipton (2006). "Activation of the Keap1/Nrf2 pathway for neuroprotection by electrophilic [correction of electrophillic] phase II inducers." *Proc Natl Acad Sci USA* 103 (3): 768-773.

Sauerbeck, A., J. Gao, R. Readnower, M. Liu, J. R. Pauly, G. Bing and P. G. Sullivan (2011). "Pioglitazone attenuates mitochondrial dysfunction, cognitive impairment, cortical tissue loss, and inflammation following traumatic brain injury." *Exp Neurol* 227 (1): 128-135.

Schaer, D. J., A. I. Alayash and P. W. Buehler (2007). "Gating the radical hemoglobin to macrophages: the anti-inflammatory role of CD163, a scavenger receptor." *Antioxid Redox Signal* 9 (7): 991-999.

Schaer, D. J., F. S. Boretti, G. Schoedon and A. Schaffner (2002). "Induction of the CD163-dependent haemoglobin uptake by macrophages as a novel anti-inflammatory action of glucocorticoids." *Br J Haematol* 119 (1): 239-243.

Schaer, D. J., F. Vinchi, G. Ingoglia, E. Tolosano and P. W. Buehler (2014). "Haptoglobin, hemopexin, and related defense pathways-basic science, clinical perspectives, and drug development." *Front Physiol* 5: 415.

Schilling, M., M. Besselmann, M. Muller, J. K. Strecker, E. B. Ringelstein and R. Kiefer (2005). "Predominant phagocytic activity of resident microglia over hematogenous macrophages following transient focal cerebral ischemia: an investigation using green fluorescent protein transgenic bone marrow chimeric mice." *Exp Neurol* 196 (2): 290-297.

Schlunk, F., E. Schulz, A. Lauer, K. Yigitkanli, W. Pfeilschifter, H. Steinmetz, E. H. Lo and C. Foerch (2015). "Warfarin pretreatment reduces cell death and MMP-9 activity in experimental intracerebral hemorrhage." *Transl Stroke Res* 6 (2): 133-139.

Servadei, F., G. Staffa, E. Pozzati and G. Piazza (1989). "Rapid spontaneous disappearance of an acute extradural hematoma: case report." *J Trauma* 29 (6): 880-882.

Sherzai, A. Z. and M. S. Elkind (2015). "Advances in stroke prevention." *Ann N Y Acad Sci* 1338: 1-15.

Shin, C. Y., M. Kundel and D. G. Wells (2004). "Rapid, activity-induced increase in tissue plasminogen activator is mediated by metabotropic glutamate receptor-dependent mRNA translation." *J Neurosci* 24 (42): 9425-9433.

Shulga, O. and N. Bornstein (2011). "Antiplatelets in secondary stroke prevention." *Front Neurol* 2: 36.

Silva, S. L., A. R. Vaz, A. Barateiro, A. S. Falcao, A. Fernandes, M. A. Brito, R. F. Silva and D. Brites (2010). "Features of bilirubin-induced reactive microglia: from phagocytosis to inflammation." *Neurobiol Dis* 40 (3): 663-675.

Silva, Y., R. Leira, J. Tejada, J. M. Lainez, J. Castillo and A. Davalos (2005). "Molecular signatures of vascular injury are associated with early growth of intracerebral hemorrhage." *Stroke* 36 (1): 86-91.

Sinha, K., J. Das, P. B. Pal and P. C. Sil (2013). "Oxidative stress: the mitochondria-dependent and mitochondria-independent pathways of apoptosis." *Arch Toxicol* 87 (7): 1157-1180.

Sinn, D. I., S. T. Lee, K. Chu, K. H. Jung, E. H. Kim, J. M. Kim, D. K. Park, E. C. Song, B. S. Kim, S. S. Yoon, M. Kim and J. K. Roh (2007). "Proteasomal inhibition in intracerebral hemorrhage: neuroprotective and anti-inflammatory effects of bortezomib." *Neurosci Res* 58 (1): 12-18.

Song, M. and S. P. Yu (2014). "Ionic regulation of cell volume changes and cell death after ischemic stroke." *Transl Stroke Res* 5 (1): 17-27.

Sorimachi, T., Y. Fujii, K. Morita and R. Tanaka (2005). "Rapid administration of antifibrinolytics and strict blood pressure control for intracerebral hemorrhage." *Neurosurgery* 57 (5): 837-844.

Stampfli, S. F., L. M. Asmis and F. C. Tanner (2008). "[Mechanism of action of old and new anticoagulants]." *Herz* 33 (1): 4-12.

Steiner, T., R. Al-Shahi Salman, R. Beer, H. Christensen, C. Cordonnier, L. Csiba, M. Forsting, S. Harnof, C. J. Klijn, D. Krieger, A. D. Mendelow, C. Molina, J. Montaner, K. Overgaard, J. Petersson, R. O. Roine, E. Schmutzhard, K. Schwerdtfeger, C. Stapf, T. Tatlisumak, B. M. Thomas, D. Toni, A. Unterberg and M. Wagner (2014). "European Stroke Organisation (ESO) guidelines for the management of spontaneous intracerebral hemorrhage." *Int J Stroke* 9 (7): 840-855.

Steiner, T. and J. Bosel (2010). "Options to restrict hematoma expansion after spontaneous intracerebral hemorrhage." *Stroke* 41 (2): 402-409.

Stoll, S., H. Hartmann, S. A. Cohen and W. E. Muller (1993). "The potent free radical scavenger alpha-lipoic acid improves memory in aged mice: putative relationship to NMDA receptor deficits." *Pharmacol Biochem Behav* 46 (4): 799-805.

Storck, S. E., S. Meister, J. Nahrath, J. N. Meissner, N. Schubert, A. Di Spiezio, S. Baches, R. E. Vandenbroucke, Y. Bouter, I. Prikulis, C. Korth, S. Weggen, A. Heimann, M. Schwaninger, T. A. Bayer and C. U. Pietrzik (2016). "Endothelial LRP1 transports amyloid-beta1-42 across the blood-brain barrier." *J Clin Invest* 126 (1): 123-136.

Stred, S. E., D. Cote, R. S. Weinstock and J. L. Messina (2003). "Regulation of hemopexin transcription by calcium ionophores and phorbol ester in hepatoma cells." *Mol Cell Endocrinol* 204 (1-2): 111-116.

Takeda, R., T. Ogura, H. Ooigawa, G. Fushihara, S. Yoshikawa, D. Okada, R. Araki and H. Kurita (2013). "A practical prediction model for early hematoma expansion in spontaneous deep ganglionic intracerebral hemorrhage." *Clin Neurol Neurosurg* 115 (7): 1028-1031.

Tejima, E., B. Q. Zhao, K. Tsuji, A. Rosell, K. van Leyen, R. G. Gonzalez, J. Montaner, X. Wang and E. H. Lo (2007). "Astrocytic induction of matrix metalloproteinase-9 and edema in brain hemorrhage." *J Cereb Blood Flow Metab* 27 (3): 460-468.

Teng, R., P. D. Mitchell and K. Butler (2014). "The effect of desmopressin on bleeding time and platelet aggregation in healthy volunteers administered ticagrelor." *J Clin Pharm Ther* 39 (2): 186-191.

Thiex, R. and S. E. Tsirka (2007). "Brain edema after intracerebral hemorrhage: mechanisms, treatment options, management strategies, and operative indications." *Neurosurg Focus* 22 (5): E6.

Tolosano, E. and F. Altruda (2002). "Hemopexin: structure, function, and regulation." *DNA Cell Biol* 21 (4): 297-306.

Tran, H. A., S. D. Chunilal and H. Tran (2014). "An update of consensus guidelines for warfarin reversal." *Med J Aust* 200 (2): 82.

Tsai, Y.-H., L.-M. Hsu, H.-H. Weng, M.-H. Lee, J.-T. Yang and C.-P. Lin (2011). "Voxel-based analysis of apparent diffusion coefficient in perihaematomal oedema: associated factors and outcome predictive value for intracerebral haemorrhage." *BMJ Open* 1 (1): e000230.

Tsivgoulis, G. and A. H. Katsanos (2015). "Intensive blood pressure reduction in acute intracerebral hemorrhage: A meta-analysis." *Neurology* 84 (24): 2464.

Tsivgoulis, G., A. H. Katsanos, K. S. Butcher, E. Boviatsis, N. Triantafyllou, I. Rizos and A. V. Alexandrov (2014). "Intensive blood pressure reduction in acute intracerebral hemorrhage: a meta-analysis." *Neurology* 83 (17): 1523-1529.

Turpie, A. G. (2008). "New oral anticoagulants in atrial fibrillation." *Eur Heart J* 29 (2): 155-165.

Valaes, T., G. S. Drummond and A. Kappas (1998). "Control of hyperbilirubinemia in glucose-6-phosphate dehydrogenase-deficient newborns using an inhibitor of bilirubin production, Sn-mesoporphyrin." *Pediatrics* 101 (5): E1.

van Aart, L., H. W. Eijkhout, J. S. Kamphuis, M. Dam, M. E. Schattenkerk, T. J. Schouten, B. Ploeger and P. F. Strengers (2006). "Individualized dosing regimen for prothrombin complex concentrate more effective than standard treatment in the reversal of oral anticoagulant therapy: an open, prospective randomized controlled trial." *Thromb Res* 118 (3): 313-320.

van Loon, J., F. Van Calenbergh, J. Goffin and C. Plets (1993). "Controversies in the management of spontaneous cerebellar haemorrhage. A consecutive series of 49 cases and review of the literature." *Acta Neurochir (Wien)* 122 (3-4): 187-193.

van Schravendijk, M. R., S. M. Handunnetti, J. W. Barnwell and R. J. Howard (1992). "Normal human erythrocytes express CD36, an adhesion molecule of monocytes, platelets, and endothelial cells." *Blood* 80 (8): 2105-2114.

Vilahur, G., B. G. Choi, M. U. Zafar, J. F. Viles-Gonzalez, D. A. Vorchheimer, V. Fuster and J. J. Badimon (2007). "Normalization of platelet reactivity in clopidogrel-treated subjects." *J Thromb Haemost* 5 (1): 82-90.

Wada, R., R. I. Aviv, A. J. Fox, D. J. Sahlas, D. J. Gladstone, G. Tomlinson and S. P. Symons (2007). "CT angiography "spot sign" predicts hematoma expansion in acute intracerebral hemorrhage." *Stroke* 38 (4): 1257-1262.

Wada, T., H. Oara, K. Watanabe, H. Kinoshita and A. Yachi (1970). "Autoradiographic study on the site of uptake of the haptoglobin-hemoglobin complex." *J Reticuloendothel Soc* 8 (2): 185-193.

Wagner, K. R. and B. E. Dwyer (2004). "Hematoma removal, heme, and heme oxygenase following hemorrhagic stroke." *Ann N Y Acad Sci* 1012: 237-251.

Wagner, K. R., Y. Hua, G. M. de Courten-Myers, J. P. Broderick, R. N. Nishimura, S. Y. Lu and B. E. Dwyer (2000). "Tin-mesoporphyrin, a potent heme oxygenase inhibitor, for treatment of intracerebral hemorrhage: in vivo and in vitro studies." *Cell Mol Biol (Noisy-le-grand)* 46 (3): 597-608.

Wagner, K. R., F. R. Sharp, T. D. Ardizzone, A. Lu and J. F. Clark (2003). "Heme and iron metabolism: role in cerebral hemorrhage." *J Cereb Blood Flow Metab* 23 (6): 629-652.

Waje-Andreassen, U., H. Naess, L. Thomassen, T. H. Maroy, K. Y. Mazengia, G. E. Eide and C. A. Vedeler (2015). "Biomarkers Related to Carotid Intima-Media Thickness and Plaques in Long-Term Survivors of Ischemic Stroke." *Transl Stroke Res* 6 (4): 276-283.

Walsh, K. B., P. Sekar, C. D. Langefeld, C. J. Moomaw, M. S. Elkind, A. K. Boehme, M. L. James, J. Osborne, K. N. Sheth, D. Woo and O. Adeoye (2015). "Monocyte Count and 30-Day Case Fatality in Intracerebral Hemorrhage." *Stroke* 46 (8): 2302-2304.

Wang, G. (2014). "The Pathogenesis of Edema and Secondary Insults after ICH."

Wang, G., W. Hu, Q. Tang, L. Wang, X. G. Sun, Y. Chen, Y. Yin, F. Xue and Z. Sun (2015). "Effect Comparison of Both Iron Chelators on Outcomes, Iron Deposit, and Iron Transporters After Intracerebral Hemorrhage in Rats." *Mol Neurobiol.*

Wang, G., A. Manaenko, A. Shao, Y. Ou, P. Yang, E. Budbazar, D. Nowrangi, J. H. Zhang and J. Tang (2016). "Low-density lipoprotein receptor-related protein-1 facilitates heme scavenging after intracerebral hemorrhage in mice." *J Cereb Blood Flow Metab.*

Wang, G., A. Shao, W. Hu, F. Xue, H. Zhao, X. Jin, G. Li, Z. Sun and L. Wang (2015). "Changes of ferrous iron and its transporters after intracerebral hemorrhage in rats." *Int J Clin Exp Pathol* 8 (9): 10671-10679.

Wang, G., Q. Yang, G. Li, L. Wang, W. Hu, Q. Tang, D. Li and Z. Sun (2011). "Time course of heme oxygenase-1 and oxidative stress after experimental intracerebral hemorrhage." *Acta Neurochir (Wien)* 153 (2): 319-325.

Wang, G. and J. Zhang (2016). "Hematoma Expansion: Clinical and Molecular Predictors and Corresponding Pharmacological Treatment." *Curr Drug Targets.*

Wang, G. H., Z. L. Jiang, Y. C. Li, X. Li, H. Shi, Y. Q. Gao, P. S. Vosler and J. Chen (2011). "Free-radical scavenger edaravone treatment confers neuroprotection against traumatic brain injury in rats." *J Neurotrauma* 28 (10): 2123-2134.

Wang, H. M., Y. X. Zhao, S. Zhang, G. D. Liu, W. Y. Kang, H. D. Tang, J. Q. Ding and S. D. Chen (2010). "PPARgamma agonist curcumin reduces the amyloid-beta-stimulated inflammatory responses in primary astrocytes." *J Alzheimers Dis* 20 (4): 1189-1199.

Wang, J. (2010). "Preclinical and clinical research on inflammation after intracerebral hemorrhage." *Prog Neurobiol* 92 (4): 463-477.

Wang, J. and S. Dore (2007). "Heme oxygenase-1 exacerbates early brain injury after intracerebral haemorrhage." *Brain* 130 (Pt 6): 1643-1652.

Wang, W. Y., M. S. Tan, J. T. Yu and L. Tan (2015). "Role of pro-inflammatory cytokines released from microglia in Alzheimer's disease." *Ann Transl Med* 3 (10): 136.

Wang, X., H. Arima, R. Al-Shahi Salman, M. Woodward, E. Heeley, C. Stapf, P. M. Lavados, T. Robinson, Y. Huang, J. Wang, C. Delcourt and C. S. Anderson (2015). "Clinical prediction algorithm (BRAIN) to determine risk of hematoma growth in acute intracerebral hemorrhage." *Stroke* 46 (2): 376-381.

Wang, X., T. Mori, T. Sumii and E. H. Lo (2002). "Hemoglobin-induced cytotoxicity in rat cerebral cortical neurons: caspase activation and oxidative stress." *Stroke* 33 (7): 1882-1888.

Wang, Y. C., Y. Zhou, H. Fang, S. Lin, P. F. Wang, R. P. Xiong, J. Chen, X. Y. Xiong, F. L. Lv, Q. L. Liang and Q. W. Yang (2014). "Toll-like receptor 2/4 heterodimer mediates inflammatory injury in intracerebral hemorrhage." *Ann Neurol* 75 (6): 876-889.

Wells, J. E., J. Biernaskie, A. Szymanska, P. H. Larsen, V. W. Yong and D. Corbett (2005). "Matrix metalloproteinase (MMP)-12 expression has a negative impact on sensorimotor function following intracerebral haemorrhage in mice." *Eur J Neurosci* 21 (1): 187-196.

Wilkinson, K. and J. El Khoury (2012). "Microglial scavenger receptors and their roles in the pathogenesis of Alzheimer's disease." *Int J Alzheimers Dis* 2012: 489456.

Wu, G. and F. P. Huang (2005). "Effects of venom defibrase on brain edema after intracerebral hemorrhage in rats." *Acta Neurochir Suppl* 95: 381-387.

Wu, H., T. Wu, M. Li and J. Wang (2012). "Efficacy of the lipid-soluble iron chelator 2,2'-dipyridyl against hemorrhagic brain injury." *Neurobiol Dis* 45 (1): 388-394.

Wu, H., R. Zhao, J. Qi, Y. Cong, D. Wang, T. Liu, Y. Gu, X. Ban and Q. Huang (2008). "The expression and the role of protease nexin-1 on brain edema after intracerebral hemorrhage." J Neurol Sci 270 (1-2): 172-183.

Wu, J., Y. Hua, R. F. Keep, T. Nakamura, J. T. Hoff and G. Xi (2003). "Iron and iron-handling proteins in the brain after intracerebral hemorrhage." *Stroke* 34 (12): 2964-2969.

Wu, J., Y. Hua, R. F. Keep, T. Schallert, J. T. Hoff and G. Xi (2002). "Oxidative brain injury from extravasated erythrocytes after intracerebral hemorrhage." *Brain Res* 953 (1-2): 45-52.

Wu, J. S., W. M. Cheung, Y. S. Tsai, Y. T. Chen, W. H. Fong, H. D. Tsai, Y. C. Chen, J. Y. Liou, S. K. Shyue, J. J. Chen, Y. E. Chen, N. Maeda, K. K. Wu and T. N. Lin (2009). "Ligand-activated peroxisome proliferator-activated receptor-gamma protects against ischemic cerebral infarction and neuronal apoptosis by 14-3-3 epsilon upregulation." *Circulation* 119 (8): 1124-1134.

Xi, G., Y. Hua, R. F. Keep, J. G. Younger and J. T. Hoff (2001). "Systemic complement depletion diminishes perihematomal brain edema in rats." *Stroke* 32 (1): 162-167.

Xi, G., Y. Hua, R. F. Keep, J. G. Younger and J. T. Hoff (2002). "Brain edema after intracerebral hemorrhage: the effects of systemic complement depletion." *Acta Neurochir Suppl* 81: 253-256.

Xi, G., R. F. Keep and J. T. Hoff (2006). "Mechanisms of brain injury after intracerebral haemorrhage." *Lancet Neurol* 5 (1): 53-63.

Xi, G., K. R. Wagner, R. F. Keep, Y. Hua, G. M. de Courten-Myers, J. P. Broderick, T. G. Brott and J. T. Hoff (1998). "Role of blood clot formation on early edema development after experimental intracerebral hemorrhage." *Stroke* 29 (12): 2580-2586.

Xing, C., K. Arai, E. H. Lo and M. Hommel (2012). "Pathophysiologic cascades in ischemic stroke." *Int J Stroke* 7 (5): 378-385.

Xiong, X. Y., J. Wang, Z. M. Qian and Q. W. Yang (2014). "Iron and intracerebral hemorrhage: from mechanism to translation." *Transl Stroke Res* 5 (4): 429-441.

Xiong, X. Y. and Q. W. Yang (2015). "Rethinking the roles of inflammation in the intracerebral hemorrhage." *Transl Stroke Res* 6 (5): 339-341.

Xue, M., Y. Fan, S. Liu, D. A. Zygun, A. Demchuk and V. W. Yong (2009). "Contributions of multiple proteases to neurotoxicity in a mouse model of intracerebral haemorrhage." *Brain* 132 (Pt 1): 26-36.

Yagami, T., K. Ueda, K. Asakura, N. Takasu, T. Sakaeda, N. Itoh, G. Sakaguchi, J. Kishino, H. Nakazato, Y. Katsuyama, T. Nagasaki, N. Okamura, Y. Hori, K. Hanasaki, A. Arimura and M. Fujimoto (2003). "Novel binding sites of 15-deoxy-Delta12,14-prostaglandin J2 in plasma membranes from primary rat cortical neurons." *Exp Cell Res* 291 (1): 212-227.

Yaghi, S., J. Dibu, E. Achi, A. Patel, R. Samant and A. Hinduja (2014). "Hematoma expansion in spontaneous intracerebral hemorrhage: predictors and outcome." *Int J Neurosci* 124 (12): 890-893.

Yaghi, S., A. Eisenberger and J. Z. Willey (2014). "Symptomatic intracerebral hemorrhage in acute ischemic stroke after thrombolysis with intravenous recombinant tissue plasminogen activator: a review of natural history and treatment." *JAMA Neurol* 71 (9): 1181-1185.

Yang, F., D. J. Haile, F. G. Berger, D. C. Herbert, E. Van Beveren and A. J. Ghio (2003). "Haptoglobin reduces lung injury associated with exposure to blood." *Am J Physiol Lung Cell Mol Physiol* 284 (2): L402-409.

Yang, L., J. Tang, Q. Chen, B. Jiang, B. Zhang, Y. Tao, L. Li, Z. Chen and G. Zhu (2015). "Hyperbaric oxygen preconditioning attenuates neuroinflammation after intracerebral hemorrhage in rats by regulating microglia characteristics." *Brain Res* 1627: 21-30.

Yang, Z., S. Zhong, Y. Liu, H. Shen and B. Yuan (2015). "Scavenger receptor SRA attenuates microglia activation and protects neuroinflammatory injury in intracerebral hemorrhage." *J Neuroimmunol* 278: 232-238.

Yao, C., G. Wei, X. C. Lu, W. Yang, F. C. Tortella and J. R. Dave (2011). "Selective brain cooling in rats ameliorates intracerebral hemorrhage and edema caused by penetrating brain injury: possible involvement of heme oxygenase-1 expression." *J Neurotrauma* 28 (7): 1237-1245.

Yao, X., F. Zhu, Z. Zhao, C. Liu, L. Luo and Z. Yin (2011). "Arctigenin enhances chemosensitivity of cancer cells to cisplatin through inhibition of the STAT3 signaling pathway." *J Cell Biochem* 112 (10): 2837-2849.

Yasaka, M., M. Oomura, K. Ikeno, H. Naritomi and K. Minematsu (2003). "Effect of prothrombin complex concentrate on INR and blood coagulation system in emergency patients treated with warfarin overdose." *Ann Hematol* 82 (2): 121-123.

Yong, W. H., M. E. Robert, D. L. Secor, T. J. Kleikamp and H. V. Vinters (1992). "Cerebral hemorrhage with biopsy-proved amyloid angiopathy." *Arch Neurol* 49 (1): 51-58.

Yoon, C., E. A. Van Niekerk, K. Henry, T. Ishikawa, S. Orita, M. H. Tuszynski and W. M. Campana (2013). "Low-density lipoprotein receptor-related protein 1 (LRP1)-dependent cell signaling promotes axonal regeneration." *J Biol Chem* 288 (37): 26557-26568.

Yuan, B., H. Shen, L. Lin, T. Su, Z. Huang and Z. Yang (2015). "Scavenger receptor SRA attenuates TLR4-induced microglia activation in intracerebral hemorrhage." *J Neuroimmunol* 289: 87-92.

Yue, T. L., H. Y. Cheng, P. G. Lysko, P. J. McKenna, R. Feuerstein, J. L. Gu, K. A. Lysko, L. L. Davis and G. Feuerstein (1992). "Carvedilol, a new vasodilator and beta adrenoceptor antagonist, is an antioxidant and free radical scavenger." *J Pharmacol Exp Ther* 263 (1): 92-98.

Zareh, M., A. Davis and S. Henderson (2011). "Reversal of warfarin-induced hemorrhage in the emergency department." *West J Emerg Med* 12 (4): 386-392.

Zhan, L., H. Zhang, Q. Zhang, C. G. Woods, Y. Chen, P. Xue, J. Dong, E. J. Tokar, Y. Xu, Y. Hou, J. Fu, K. Yarborough, A. Wang, W. Qu, M. P. Waalkes, M. E. Andersen and J. Pi (2012). "Regulatory role of KEAP1 and NRF2 in PPARgamma expression and chemoresistance in human non-small-cell lung carcinoma cells." *Free Radic Biol Med* 53 (4): 758-768.

Zhang, H., Y. J. Su, W. W. Zhou, S. W. Wang, P. X. Xu, X. L. Yu and R. T. Liu (2014). "Activated scavenger receptor A promotes glial internalization of abeta." *PLoS One* 9 (4): e94197.

Zhang, L., D. Johnson and J. A. Johnson (2013). "Deletion of Nrf2 impairs functional recovery, reduces clearance of myelin debris and decreases axonal remyelination after peripheral nerve injury." *Neurobiol Dis* 54: 329-338.

Zhao, H., S. Hao, H. Xu, L. Ma, Z. Zhang, Y. Ni and L. Yu (2016). "Protective role of nuclear factor erythroid 2-related factor 2 in the hemorrhagic shock-induced inflammatory response." *Int J Mol Med* 37 (4): 1014-1022.

Zhao, X. and J. Aronowski (2013). "Nrf2 to pre-condition the brain against injury caused by products of hemolysis after ICH." *Transl Stroke Res* 4 (1): 71-75.

Zhao, X., J. Grotta, N. Gonzales and J. Aronowski (2009). "Hematoma resolution as a therapeutic target: the role of microglia/macrophages." *Stroke 40 (3 Suppl):* S92-94.

Zhao, X., S. Song, G. Sun, R. Strong, J. Zhang, J. C. Grotta and J. Aronowski (2009). "Neuroprotective role of haptoglobin after intracerebral hemorrhage." *J Neurosci* 29 (50): 15819-15827.

Zhao, X., S. Song, G. Sun, J. Zhang, R. Strong, L. Zhang, J. C. Grotta and J. Aronowski (2011). "Cytoprotective role of haptoglobin in brain after experimental intracerebral hemorrhage." *Acta Neurochir Suppl* 111: 107-112.

Zhao, X., R. Strong, J. Zhang, G. Sun, J. Z. Tsien, Z. Cui, J. C. Grotta and J. Aronowski (2009). "Neuronal PPARgamma deficiency increases susceptibility to brain damage after cerebral ischemia." *J Neurosci* 29 (19): 6186-6195.

Zhao, X., G. Sun, S. M. Ting, S. Song, J. Zhang, N. J. Edwards and J. Aronowski (2015). "Cleaning up after ICH: the role of Nrf2 in modulating microglia function and hematoma clearance." *J Neurochem* 133 (1): 144-152.

Zhao, X., G. Sun, J. Zhang, R. Strong, W. Song, N. Gonzales, J. C. Grotta and J. Aronowski (2007). "Hematoma resolution as a target for intracerebral hemorrhage treatment: role for peroxisome proliferator-activated receptor gamma in microglia/macrophages." *Ann Neurol* 61 (4): 352-362.

Zhao, X., Y. Zhang, R. Strong, J. C. Grotta and J. Aronowski (2006). "15d-Prostaglandin J2 activates peroxisome proliferator-activated receptor-gamma, promotes expression of catalase, and reduces inflammation, behavioral dysfunction, and neuronal loss after intracerebral hemorrhage in rats." *J Cereb Blood Flow Metab* 26 (6): 811-820.

Zhao, X. R., N. Gonzales and J. Aronowski (2015). "Pleiotropic role of PPARgamma in intracerebral hemorrhage: an intricate system involving Nrf2, RXR, and NF-kappaB." *CNS Neurosci Ther* 21 (4): 357-366.

Zhao, Y., A. Patzer, T. Herdegen, P. Gohlke and J. Culman (2006). "Activation of cerebral peroxisome proliferator-activated receptors gamma promotes neuroprotection by attenuation of neuronal cyclooxygenase-2 overexpression after focal cerebral ischemia in rats." *Faseb j* 20 (8): 1162-1175.

Zhou, W., S. Schwarting, S. Illanes, A. Liesz, M. Middelhoff, M. Zorn, M. Bendszus, S. Heiland, J. van Ryn and R. Veltkamp (2011). "Hemostatic therapy in experimental intracerebral hemorrhage associated with the direct thrombin inhibitor dabigatran." *Stroke* 42 (12): 3594-3599.

Zhou, W., M. Zorn, P. Nawroth, U. Butehorn, E. Perzborn, S. Heitmeier and R. Veltkamp (2013). "Hemostatic therapy in experimental intracerebral hemorrhage associated with rivaroxaban." *Stroke* 44 (3): 771-778.

Zhou, X., Q. Xie, G. Xi, R. F. Keep and Y. Hua (2014). "Brain CD47 Expression in a Swine Model of Intracerebral Hemorrhage." *Brain research* 1574: 70-76.

Zhou, Y., Y. Wang, J. Wang, R. Anne Stetler and Q. W. Yang (2014). "Inflammation in intracerebral hemorrhage: from mechanisms to clinical translation." *Prog Neurobiol* 115: 25-44.

Zielinski, I. M., M. L. Jongsma, C. M. Baas, P. B. Aarts and B. Steenbergen (2014). "Unravelling developmental disregard in children with unilateral cerebral palsy by measuring event-related potentials during a simple and complex task." *BMC Neurol* 14: 6.

Zlokovic, B. V. (2010). "Neurodegeneration and the neurovascular unit." *Nat Med* 16 (12): 1370-1371.

Zuwala-Jagiello, J. (2006). "Haemoglobin scavenger receptor: function in relation to disease." *Acta Biochim Pol* 53 (2): 257-268.

ABOUT THE AUTHOR

Gaiqing Wang

Associate Professor of Neurology
Clinical Educator, Master's supervisor
Department of Neurology,
The second hospital of Shanxi Medical University,
Taiyuan, Shanxi, China
E-mail: wanggq08@126.com

Research interests: The brain injury after intracerebral hemorrhage

Education:

- 1988.8-1993.7: B.M. Major in Clinical Medicine, Shanxi Medical College; Taiyuan, China ,
- 1999.9-2002.7: M.M. Major in Child psychology, Shanxi Medical University; Taiyuan, China ,
- 2003.9-2006.7: M.D. Major in Neurology, XiangYa Medical College of Central-South University, Changsha, China
- 2014.9-2015.9: Postdoc. Major in Neuroscience, Loma Linda University, Loma Linda, 92354, CA, US

Representative Publications:

1. Gaiqing Wang and John H. Zhang. Hematoma Expansion: Clinical and Molecular Predictors and Corresponding Pharmacological Treatment. Curr Drug Targets. 2016 Jul 11. [Epub ahead of print]

2. Low-density lipoprotein receptor-related protein-1 Facilitates Heme Scavenging after Intracerebral Hemorrhage in Mice. J Cereb Blood Flow Metab. 2016
3. Effect Comparison of Both Iron Chelators on Outcomes, Iron Deposit, and Iron Transporters After Intracerebral Hemorrhage in Rats. Mol Neurobiol. 2015
4. Changes of Ferrous Iron and Its Transporters after Intracerebral Hemorrhage in Rats. Int J Clin Exp Pathol. 2015
5. The Pathogenesis of Edema and Secondary Insults after ICH. Intracerebral hemorrhage.Dr. Vikas Chaudhary (Ed.), ISBN: 978-953-51-1722-3, InTech, 2014;
6. Time course of heme oxygenase-1 and oxidative stress after experimental intracerebral hemorrhage. Acta Neurochir. 2011
7. Brain edema after intracerebral hemorrhage in rats: the role of iron overload and aquaporin 4. J Neurosurg. 2009

INDEX

D

E

F

G

H

I

J

K

L

M

R

S

T

U

V

W

Y

Z